# Effects of Antenatal Exercise on Psychological Well-being, Pregnancy and Birth Outcome

# Effects of Antenatal Exercise on Psychological Well-being, Pregnancy and Birth Outcome

## Jean Rankin

PhD, MSc, BSc (Hons), RM, RGN, RSCN, PGCE
University of Paisley

WHURR
PUBLISHERS

© 2002 Whurr Publishers Ltd
First published 2002 by
Whurr Publishers Ltd
19b Compton Terrace
London N1 2UN, England, and 325 Chestnut Street,
Philadelphia PA 19106, USA

**British Library Cataloguing in Publication Data**
A catalogue record for this book is available from the
British Library.

ISBN 1 86156 292 6

# Contents

# Foreword

Exercise during pregnancy has an intriguing history as readers of this book will no doubt find out. In the 17th and 18th century exercise was encouraged to ensure good health and to prevent miscarriage but a century later the pregnant mothers were advised not to do anything strenuous in order to guard against ligament strain and prolapse of the womb. Today most people are aware of the value of regular activity for health but myths and mysteries still surround the topic of exercise during pregnancy. This book should help dispel such myths, and offers professionals and pregnant women evidence-based advice about what kind of exercise should be undertaken, the benefits that might be realised and contraindications to be aware of. The specific contributions this book makes include a history of exercise in pregnancy, a review of the beneficial effects of exercise, a discussion of psychological aspects of pregnancy (which are often neglected) and practical guidelines for professionals to follow when they are advising pregnant women about exercise.

Jean Rankin is extremely well qualified to write on this topic. She has over twenty years experience as a practising midwife and in between times she has found the time and energy to complete BSc, MSc and PhD degrees from Glasgow University. Each of these degrees extended her knowledge of how exercise can be a useful aspect of antenatal care, and her PhD examined exactly what happens to women who exercise during pregnancy . The results of that work in Chapter 4 show a very positive picture of exercise helping women maintain prepregnancy levels of mood.

Jean is one of the very few people who have conducted well designed research in this area. She is also able to influence the training and practice of midwifery from her position as Senior Lecturer at Paisley University. It has been my privilege to be involved in the supervision of Jean's academic work. She was a student with a passion to connect her knowledge of exercise science to the profession of midwifery. She dedicated a substantial part of her life to this process simultaneously juggling family, work and study commitments in a way that often left me in awe of her energy. This book shows that all of that effort was worthwhile; it will be useful for midwives, student nurses, obstetricians, exercise scientists and fitness professionals. This work will make a significant impact in the field of exercise science and in the profession of midwifery, and should encourage the notion that exercise should be a normal part of antenatal care.

Nanette Mutrie
Professor of Physical Activity and Health Science
University of Glasgow
January 2002

# Preface

The study and PhD thesis on which this book is based derived from my work as a midwife with a special interest in exercise. The study was originally an idea that just kept recurring. Eventually, I was encouraged to take the initial step to plan this venture that was to take five years to complete. The research was undertaken as a part-time PhD and I continued to work full time initially as a senior midwife then as a midwifery lecturer. The first two years of the study were self-funded and thereafter I secured funding from Ayrshire and Arran Health Board for the women in the study and funding from North Ayrshire and Arran NHS Trust to set up the exercise class. The University of Paisley partially funded my final year of PhD study.

The main aims of the study were to investigate the effects of a regular exercise programme during and after pregnancy on psychological well-being, pregnancy and birth outcomes. The aims were met using a randomized control trial of healthy primigravid women assigned to either a control group or an intervention group. The control group continued with the existing antenatal education programme and, in addition to this, the intervention group participated in an antenatal exercise programme. Subjects were recruited at the first antenatal appointment in early pregnancy and continued until 16 weeks postpartum. Of the subjects ($n$ = 157) recruited, 98 (62%) completed the study, of whom 48 (49%) were in the control group and 50 (51%) in the intervention group.

Data were collected at three time points during and after pregnancy using a variety of outcome measures, and were analysed using appropriate statistical testing. Conclusions were drawn indicating that women who participated in regular physical activity tended to have protection against reduction of psychological well-being, as measured by a variety of psychological constructs. The maintenance in psychological well-being was experienced both during and after pregnancy, and there was no indication of any risk to the pregnancy or the baby. This was in contrast to the significant reduction in psychological well-being experienced by the women in the control group during the same period. No differences were found between the groups in relation to pregnancy and birth outcomes. All births had a positive outcome and were uncomplicated.

This book takes the reader through each stage of the study, from planning to completion, and recommendations for practice and further research. I have attempted to make this study as interesting and readable as possible, but it was necessary to include some of the more intricate statistical findings. This was my first attempt at a major study and it was not plain sailing. On hindsight, I have learned a lot and I was privileged to be part of this special time in the women's lives.

Pregnancy is a time when women need to be prepared mentally and physically to meet the challenges of childbirth and the transition to parenthood. However, this needs to be within the realms of safe practice. It is hoped that readers, particularly those involved in some capacity with women during pregnancy, will be encouraged to undertake similar work in this field of interest.

# Acknowledgements

I would like to thank the following people:

My supervisors at the University of Glasgow, Professor Nanette Mutrie and Professor Edith Hillan, for their guidance, continued support, constructive feedback and encouragement during this study.

Mr Tom Aitchison, Statistics Department, University of Glasgow, for statistical support.

Midwives, obstetricians and physiotherapists, for their contribution during the planning of the study.

Midwifery friends and colleagues who offered continued support and encouragement.

All the women who participated in the study and were a joy to work with.

London Central YMCA who provided exercise instructors' training.

Ayrshire and Arran Health Board, University of Paisley, and North Ayrshire and Arran NHS Trust who provided funding.

On a more personal note:

I am privileged to have special friends: Avis, for her support and encouragement every step of the way, and Marta: '*Secundas res splendidiores facit amicitia.*'

Nanette Mutrie who had faith in me to take this study one step further.

Special thanks to Louise and Martin for their encouragement, and keeping my midwifery skills updated by having four children during the study and baby number five during the writing of this book.

To Lynsay and Lee, my children, who have developed into bright and intelligent young adults. This is a gift to you both.

Finally, I dedicate this book to my mum and dad without whose love, support and encouragement this endeavour would not have been possible.

# Glossary of terms

**Abortion:** this is the term used to denote an interruption of pregnancy before week 24 of gestation.

**Aerobic capacity (VO$_2$)** refers to the rate at which oxygen can be used by the cells. It can be described as absolute or functional aerobic capacity. The evaluation of *functional* aerobic capacity describes the individual's capacity to meet and sustain daily weight-bearing activities whereas *absolute* aerobic capacity is a measure of the individual's maximal cardiopulmonary capacity and maximal energy output by aerobic processes.

**Anoxia** refers to the lack of oxygen which, if it persists, will result in death of the fetus.

**Apgar score** is a numerical assessment of the newborn in terms of general condition immediately after birth. This involves consideration of the degree to which the following five signs are present or absent: heart rate, respiratory effort, muscle tone, reflex and colour.

**Birthweight** is the first weight of the newborn obtained preferably within 1 hour of birth before significant postnatal weight loss has occurred.

**Bradycardia** is fetal heart rate below 120 beats/min.

**Cardiotocography** is the use of Doppler ultrasonography to make an immediate assessment of fetoplacental well-being. This is provided by a trace of the fetal heart rate (cardio) in relation to the activity and pressure in the uterus (toco).

**Congenital abnormalities** refers to any abnormalities present at birth.

**Contracted pelvis** refers to a pelvis with all diameters reduced by 1 cm.

**Duration of labour** averages between 10 and 12 hours for a primigravida and 6 hours for a multigravida.

**Dystocia** is the term used to encompass all the factors that cause labour to be prolonged. The term 'dystocia' originates from the Greek words '*Dys*' meaning 'bad or abnormal' and '*Tokos*' meaning 'labour'.

**Episiotomy** refers to the surgical incision of the perineum and vagina, which enlarges the introitus to facilitate delivery of the baby.

**Fetus** is the term used to describe the human being from week 10 of gestation until birth.

**Fetal** refers to the fetus.

**Fetal bradycardia** refers to the fetal heart rate of less than 120 beats/min. Marked bradycardia is a fetal heart rate of less than 100 beats/min.

**Fetal tachycardia** refers to the fetal heart rate greater than 160 beats/min.

**Gestation of pregnancy** is the period of gestation calculated from the date of the last menstrual period and normally is of 40 weeks' duration. *Gestational age* of the pregnancy or fetus refers to this period.

**Gravid** is the term used for pregnant, e.g. gravid uterus.

**Hypertension** refers to blood pressure of greater than 140/90 mmHg or a rise of between 15 and 20 mmHg in the systolic pressure and between 10 and 15 mmHg in the diastolic pressure.

**Hypoxia** refers to a lack of oxygen that can result in distress of the fetus *in utero*.

**Labour** refers to the process by which the fetus, placenta and membranes are expelled through the birth canal. There are three stages of labour. The first stage is passive and begins from the onset of regular, rhythmic uterine contractions until full dilatation of the cervix, the second stage is defined from full dilatation of the cervix until delivery of the baby and the third stage occurs from delivery of the baby until expulsion of the placenta and membranes.

**Late deceleration** refers to a drop in fetal heart rate, which shows the lowest level of deceleration lagging behind the highest peak of the uterine contraction.

**Low birthweight** is a birthweight of less than 2500 grams. This includes pre-term infants and growth-retarded infants of maturity more than 37 weeks.

**Maximal oxygen consumption** ($VO_{2max}$) is defined as the maximal rate at which oxygen can be used by the cells in the body. It is a non-invasive measurement of physical fitness, which is a measure of cardiovascular endurance. This includes a circulatory component to oxygen uptake (*oxygen delivery*) and an extraction component (*oxygen utilization*).

**Multigravida** is the term used for a woman who is pregnant for the second or subsequent time.

**Neonatal** is the term used for the newborn infant (neonate) in the first 28 days of life.

**Neonatal period** describes the first 28 days of life.

**Normal labour** is a labour in which the fetus presents by the vertex, the occiput rotates anteriorly and the result is the birth of a living, mature fetus with no complications, the duration of labour ranging from 4 to 24 hours.

**Obstructed labour** is the term used to describe labour when there is no descent of the presenting part in the presence of good contractions. Usually there is extensive caput and moulding, and malposition or malpresentation. The fetus is often large and the pelvis small or abnormal in shape.

**Occiput** is the term used to describe the back of the fetal head behind the posterior fontanelle.

**Operative delivery** is normally by lower uterine segment caesarean section (LUSCS), which is the surgical removal of the fetus by the abdominal route after fetal viability (week 24).

**Partum** is the term used to refer to the period of childbirth. *Antepartum* refers to the period before labour and delivery, *intrapartum* refers to the period during labour and delivery and *postpartum* refers to the 6-week period after delivery.

**Placenta** is the organ of communication between the fetus and the mother. This provides the blood supply with nutrition and products of metabolism.

**Postnatal period** refers to the first 28 days after delivery of the baby.

**Precipitous labour** describes labour that is very rapid with intense frequent contractions, which results in the delivery of the baby within 1 hour.

**Pre-term baby** refers to a baby born before the 37th completed week of pregnancy.

**Pre-term delivery** refers to labour and delivery occurring before the completion of week 37 of pregnancy.

**Primigravida** is the term used to describe a woman who is pregnant for the first time.

**Spontaneous vertex delivery (SVD)** refers to the normal delivery of the baby. The fetus is described as being a cephalic presentation and longitudinal lie with a well-flexed head. The fetus negotiates the pelvis and is delivered vaginally. The vertex refers to the area of the fetal skull bounded by the parietal eminences and the anterior and posterior fontanelles.

# Chapter 1
# Introduction

## Background

Exercise is now universally advocated as a means to maintain and enhance good physical and mental health. In fact, there is general agreement that regular exercise by healthy individuals has psychological and physical benefits that include improved physical fitness and enhanced quality of life (Griffiths 1996). More recently, these benefits are acknowledged in national strategies that aim to promote regular physical activity in the general population, with women of all ages identified as one of the target groups (Scottish Office Home and Health Department 1992; Royal College of Physicians 1993).

Women today are more autonomous and feel empowered to be in control of their health, mind and body, and for many women exercise has become an integral part of normal life. Over recent decades, the increasing trend for exercise is reflected in the number of pregnant women who are also adopting a more active lifestyle (Artal and Sherman 1999; Clapp 2000).

Many women may participate in physical activity for recreation, health benefits or as part of a fitness or training programme. More often, women regularly participate in exercise as part of an exercise-related career or to enhance sports performance. Information has consistently suggested that exercise may be particularly beneficial for women (Berger 1984; Tanji 2000). Several reviews have suggested that exercise can be beneficial in helping women cope with issues faced in reproductive life (Gannon 1988; Choi and Mutrie 1996).

Most exercising women wish to remain physically active during pregnancy so that they can continue to enjoy the physical and psychological benefits (Halksworth 1993). In particular, there has been a growing demand for exercise, specifically for pregnant women who are not accustomed to exercise but who wish to exercise in order to take better care of themselves and their babies during pregnancy (Gaskill 1993; Mottola and Wolfe 1994).

1

Pregnancy is a very special time in a woman's life and pregnant women are concerned for their own health and fitness and also about doing what is best for the health of the baby (Horns et al. 1996). Some women may be reluctant to start or continue to exercise during pregnancy for fear of harming their unborn baby (Halksworth 1993). Women want to learn all they can about remaining active during pregnancy, what potential benefits and risks there are in pregnancy, how much exercise is safe for the baby, and how pregnancy will affect their sports performance (Artal Mittlemark et al. 1991a). Therefore it is to be expected that more women will now be approaching health professionals for advice and guidance about exercise during pregnancy. Women should be given sound advice based on evidence to enable them to continue to exercise safely and confidently during pregnancy.

There are also important fundamental questions of interest to health professionals and exercise scientists. These include the ways in which pregnancy alters the woman's ability to exercise, to what extent the response to exercise during pregnancy differs from that in the non-pregnant state, and in what way physical activity influences the course of pregnancy and the development of the fetus (Artal Mittlemark et al. 1991a; Mottola and Wolfe 1994). Pregnancy is one of the life events that provides an opportunity to promote a healthy lifestyle. This 'health-promoting' opportunity may be lost if there is a lack of knowledge and understanding in the area of exercise during pregnancy.

The impact of pregnancy and childbirth presents physical and psychological challenges to women. The process of childbirth itself has been depicted as a normal developmental positive experience (Zajicek 1981; McGoldrick and Carter 1982). Others have described pregnancy as a developmental or maturational crisis involving one of the greatest transitions in a woman's life (Bibring 1959; Erikson 1965; Grossman et al. 1980). Therefore, any physical or psychological benefits gained through exercise would be an advantage to pregnant women during this important life event.

Pregnancy is probably one of the most important times in a woman's life it is desirable that exercise is carried out safely and correctly. However, the unique physical and physiological conditions that exist during pregnancy and the postpartum period create special risks that do not affect non-pregnant women (Kramer 2000). Careful consideration should be given to the additional impact that exercise may have on the progressive anatomical, physiological and psychological changes that normally occur during pregnancy (Artal Mittlemark et al. 1991a; Wells 1991).

In general, there appears to be no contraindication to exercise during pregnancy in the healthy woman (Wells 1991). In fact, there is belief in the value of safe exercise during pregnancy, provided that any advice given is appropriate to the needs of the individual woman (Huch and Erkkola 1990; Lokey et al. 1991; Clapp 2000; Kramer 2000). The course and outcome of pregnancy are much influenced by general health and lifestyle. Effort is now being put into educating both potential parents to 'get fit for pregnancy'. Exercise provides a sense of well-being and accomplishment and improves physical fitness (Cowlin 1997). There is no doubt that improved stamina, well-being and self-reliance would benefit women in their preparation for the physical and emotional challenges inherent in pregnancy and childbirth, and in the transition to parenthood (Artal and Artal Mittlemark 1991).

It is important that up-to-date scientific research is available to support existing findings on the effects of exercise during pregnancy. Information, based on sound research findings, should be widely disseminated and readily available to health professionals concerned with pregnant women. This would allow the health professionals to provide up-to-date, accurate and appropriate advice and guidance to pregnant women. Possible benefits and available opportunities to gain these benefits should be incorporated into antenatal education programmes to enable women to make informed choices and be supported if they wish to exercise during and after pregnancy.

## The development of the researcher's interest in exercise and pregnancy

As the researcher I have two main interests in life that form the basis for this study. As a midwife, I am very much involved with women during pregnancy and in the transition to parenthood. This is a normal life event and women should have every opportunity and support to make this a positive experience. I have enjoyed an active lifestyle and my life is enriched with the many benefits gained over the years.

Some 20 years ago, it seemed natural for me to continue with my active lifestyle during pregnancy. However, at the time there was little or no support offered by the health professionals, and it was frowned upon that I even considered putting myself and my baby at risk. I did continue to exercise regularly with modifications but decided to keep this information from the experts. On hindsight, this was not a good idea and most definitely not to be recommended.

This attitude towards women and exercise continued during the 1980s. As both a midwife and exerciser, I often met women in similar circumstances and dilemmas about exercising during pregnancy. It was a fact of life that some women continued to exercise despite the lack of support and information. This was evident with the number of pregnant women attending general exercise classes. There was no doubt that the women were enjoying themselves. I was, however, concerned that the exercise was often undertaken with incorrect technique and little guidance related to the changes of pregnancy.

At this time, Nanette Mutrie, Senior Lecturer in Sports Science at the University of Glasgow, advised me to 'do something about it'. This advice was the impetus for a radical change in attitudes and practice. Aquanatal classes were set up in local health centres by me and this quickly gained momentum. It was not all plain sailing, but support was on the increase. By 1990, aquanatal classes were established in most local areas and these were run by 'suitably trained' midwives and exercise instructors. Many health professionals remained sceptical and often quoted the lack of evidence in favour of supportive anecdotal information. I then decided to review the available literature. I was inspired by the work undertaken by the London Central YMCA and enlightened to discover how much more advanced other countries were in this field. It was at this point that I decided to undertake this study.

The planning stage began in 1994 and this was only the beginning of a five-year journey. The first priority was to design a study that addressed some gaps in the existing literature but remained within the capacity of a single researcher. The study was a two-group, randomized controlled study of healthy women during their first pregnancy. The control group continued with the existing antenatal preparation of women for pregnancy, childbirth and the transition to parenthood. In addition, the intervention group participated in a regular structured 'antenatal and postnatal exercise programme'. Participants were recruited in early pregnancy and continued in the study until 4 months after delivery.

The study became of interest to women, midwives, other health professionals and exercise instructors at a local level. As a result, I am delighted to report that positive changes have taken place in the attitude to both exercise in pregnancy and the provision of services offered to women in the local area. This book takes the reader through each stage of the study from planning to completion.

## Plan of the book

This first chapter provides an overview of the current situation where exercise is now promoted as a means of gaining physical, psychological and health benefits. There has been a recent trend for more women to exercise regularly and this includes women who want to exercise during pregnancy. The special risks created by the physical and physiological changes of pregnancy make this an important time when exercise is carried out safely and correctly. In this respect, the interest and concerns of women themselves, health professionals and exercise scientists, in relation to the effect that exercise may have on pregnancy and birth outcome and well-being of the baby, are identified.

The background to the study from a personal perspective is presented. This details my personal and professional experience of exercise, pregnancy, and exercise during and after pregnancy. This experience was the impetus for the present study with a view to contributing evidence to the existing body of literature in this field of interest.

Chapter 2 presents a review of the psychological and physiological changes of pregnancy. In particular, there is a focus on the progressive anatomical and physiological changes of pregnancy, which need to be considered in the context of exercise having a further impact on pregnancy. An overview of the physiological, psychological and potential health benefits of exercise to the non-pregnant population is presented. This is followed by an overview of exercise in obstetrics from an historical perspective. Thereafter, there is a detailed review of the current literature in relation to scientific evidence of the physiological and psychological effects of exercise on pregnancy, birth outcomes and the postpartum period. The review highlights gaps in the existing literature and research methodologies, the basis for the present study and issues for future research. The present study is discussed in terms of the need for research in this area and the aims and objectives of the research.

Chapter 3 defines the methodology and theoretical approach to the study. The methods are discussed in detail, and justification for the design is presented. The pilot study is presented, because it was an important prelude to the methodology used in the main study. The exercise programme is detailed in relation to the components of the programme, the underlying principles based on the physiological changes of pregnancy, and exercise guidelines adhered to during the study and the current guidelines for exercise in pregnancy.

Chapter 4 reports the findings and contains detailed analyses of the data obtained. This section is subdivided into the findings related to: demographic details, psychological indicators of well-being, pregnancy and birth outcomes, physical activity details, and pregnancy and birth outcomes for those participants who dropped out of the study.

Chapter 5 contains a detailed synthesis of the findings from the study in relation to psychological indicators, pregnancy and birth outcomes, and physical activity outcomes. The relevance of these findings to current knowledge is discussed.

Chapter 6 presents the conclusions and recommendations for practice based on the findings from the study. The recommendations for further research in this area of interest are presented.

The Appendices provide additional detailed information about issues presented and discussed within the book.

# Chapter 2
# Review of the literature

This chapter provides a review of the literature relevant to exercise and pregnancy. The reader will note the length and diversity of the review, and it is important to clarify the reasons for this.

First, both pregnancy and exercise are reviewed separately. This was designed to allow the reader to gain an insight into each area of interest before the impact of exercise on pregnancy was reviewed. Second, there is an overview of the literature from an historical perspective. The purpose of this was to present the reader with background reading of women and society and the association between pregnancy and physical activity throughout recognized periods of history. This section takes the reader through the different perceptions and attitudes towards women, pregnancy and physical activity, and the associated developments in practice to the modern day.

Third, there is a review of the scientific investigations of exercise and pregnancy over the previous 30 years. This review and exploration was an important prerequisite to undertaking the present study. The final section presents a summary of the gaps in the literature and the purpose of the present study. The basis for the present study was to address relevant issues and gaps identified from previous research within the research design. The reader should note that a single researcher undertook the present study. Subsequently, this was reflected in the research design and credence was given only to those issues that could be appropriately addressed within the research design.

The review has four distinct but associated sections that will take the reader through the various elements leading to the main study:

1. The impact of pregnancy and childbirth presents psychological, physical and physiological challenges to women. The psychological changes occurring during pregnancy and childbirth are presented, in addition to the physical and physiological changes that can influ-ence the effects of exercise. These unique changes create special

risks during exercise that do not affect non-pregnant women. Exercise has many connotations to individuals and there is an explanation of associated terminology used. An overview of the benefits of exercise to the healthy individual is presented in relation to the physical, psychological and health benefits associated with regular exercise and the mechanisms proposed for psychological benefits.

2. An historical overview of the literature is detailed from biblical times through to twentieth century practice. This section presents the literature available over each era in relation to attitudes, perceptions associated with women, society, pregnancy and physical activity. Developments in the advice and support given to women about exercise and pregnancy over the different historical periods are presented.

3. A review of the scientific investigation of the literature over the previous 30 years is presented. To date, there is a wealth of literature available on the physiological effects of exercise on pregnancy. For the purpose of this study, a summarized review of these findings is presented. A detailed review is presented in relation to pregnancy and birth outcomes and the psychological effects of exercise during pregnancy.

4. This section highlights the gaps in the existing literature and the subsequent areas of interest; methodological issues are identified that are addressed in the present study. The purpose of the present study is detailed.

# Changes of pregnancy

## Psychological factors

Pregnancy is generally regarded as a critical event in a woman's life. The psychological changes occurring during pregnancy and early motherhood are rapid when compared with other periods in adult life. Some of the changes may only be temporary as a result of biological events and other factors, whereas other changes may be more long-term and affect psychological well-being. The physical and mental events during childbirth affect one another intimately.

The psychological effects of pregnancy have been of interest for many years and the literature presents conflicting accounts of women's experiences of pregnancy. Although some studies present pregnancy as being a normal and positive maturing experience (Zajicek 1981; Osofsky and Osofsky 1984), others depict pregnancy as a psychological and biological crisis (Bibring 1959; Grossman et al. 1980). A variety of theoretical views has been put forward concerning the psychological and emotional aspects of pregnancy. Deutsch (1947) describes pregnancy as a calm dream-like period that fulfils a woman's deepest yearnings. Conversely, Bibring (1959) views pregnancy as inherently a period of emotional, psychological and social stress, with the level of anxiety increasing as pregnancy progresses (Bibring et al. 1961).

The emotional reactions to pregnancy play an important part in everyday obstetric and midwifery practice. Many factors influence and determine a woman's reactions to pregnancy and how she will eventually cope with her feelings about the pregnancy, birth and transition to parenthood. Although every woman is unique, emotional and cognitive reactions are found to be common. These include anxiety, hostility, fatigue, introversion, mood swings, denial and impatience (Chalmers 1982). Negative changes in body image are common because pregnancy alters the body shape and size (Strang and Sullivan 1985).

Social and cultural factors strongly influence the woman's perception of pregnancy (Price 1993a). The interaction between the physiological changes of pregnancy, personality, lifestyle, relationships, health and fitness status, feelings about herself and having a baby will, to a large extent, influence the woman's perception of pregnancy.

The anxiety experienced by women during pregnancy has been related to the trimester of pregnancy (Friederich 1977; Pitt 1977). Findings from empirical studies indicate that women tend to feel both happy and anxious in early pregnancy (Green 1990a). Pregnant women report increased levels of anxiety, depression and irritability when compared with the non-pregnant state (Condon 1987). Green (1990b) reported that some women tend to be preoccupied with worry from early pregnancy onwards about various aspects of pregnancy. Negative feelings, particularly related to the birth, were found to peak around the third trimester of pregnancy (Elliot et al. 1983). However, some women may never experience these negative emotions and increased levels of psychological well-being have actually been reported (Elliot et al. 1983; Condon 1987).

The individual coping style of women may determine the level of self-esteem and sense of achievement felt as pregnancy progresses. The literature indicates that the symptoms reported are associated with negative attitudes towards pregnancy, particularly in the later stages. The results of empirical research indicate that pregnancy is not entirely pleasurable for most women. Wolkind and Zajicek (1981) reported that physical discomforts were common during pregnancy with emotional events such as crying, worry, misery and nervousness being common in the second and early third trimesters. Women who were highly distressed, anxious or depressed during pregnancy were found to be more likely to experience depression in the postnatal period (Elliot et al. 1983; Watson et al. 1984; Sharp 1989). These high levels of stress and distress can have an adverse effect on both the fetus and the relationship that the mother has with her partner, friends and family. Green (1990a) suggests that the mood of women in the antenatal period is an important predictor of the mood in the postnatal period.

Glazer (1980) recommended that it was important to reduce the levels of maternal anxiety to improve the pregnant woman's emotional and physical well-being and protect the fetus. The emotional states of the mother during pregnancy affect the delivery process. In particular, a high level of maternal anxiety is associated with a variety of obstetric complications, including prolonged labour and births. Findings such as these have contributed to the development of antenatal programmes that aim to enhance the emotional state of women and improve their attitude towards childbirth.

Outward acceptance or even enthusiasm for the pregnancy may conceal anxiety and fear. Even when the woman views pregnancy as highly desirable, there are unavoidable tensions between her perceived personal needs and desires and the growing fetus. These may include the pregnancy perceived as an invasion of privacy or an intrusion in personal relationships, an alteration to lifestyle, and a loss of career opportunities or independence. The changing roles experienced by women may be in conflict and be associated with a loss of control (Ball 1989; Price 1993b). The pregnant woman may feel that she is perceived as a 'pregnancy' only and that her identity becomes submerged (Alder 1994).

Natural life processes such as adolescence and pregnancy represent a normal body image adjustment for women. The individual's image of her body arises from formulated opinion and feelings through visual assessment of body appearance and sensations (Ussher 1993). Pregnancy radically alters the physical dimensions and function of the body and a woman's sense of completeness and sexual identity (Price 1996). The body image associated with pregnancy, childbirth and breast-feeding involves a significant distortion of the woman's normal body contours, her weight and body sensations. The woman's perception of body reality is set against an 'ideal body' and this will be different for each woman. The woman can either accept that the pregnant woman 'blooms' or cause the woman to lament the loss of a smaller, thinner appearance (Price 1993a). Pregnancy poses a more significant challenge to the woman's perception of her body than any other body adjustments (Price 1993a, 1993b, 1996).

Changing body image in pregnancy can have a powerful effect on a woman and her partner (Sweet and Tiran 1997). These may be either positive or negative changes and can extend to affect sexual and postpartum relationships between the woman and her partner (Price 1993b). The adjustment to pregnancy might be dominated by the woman's developing relationship with her baby, with her relationship to the baby's father taking second place. There is evidence to associate the quality of marital relationships with the psychological well-being of the mother during pregnancy. Scott-Heyes (1984) suggests that women are more likely to suffer from depression if they have poor marital relationships during pregnancy.

There are a variety of interpersonal, cultural and physical challenges confronting the woman and her partner during pregnancy, childbirth and parenthood. These all occur for the couple within a compact timeframe which also needs to incorporate their individual sexual identity and shared relationship. The literature agrees that a woman's level of sexual interest changes during pregnancy and remains altered for weeks or months after the birth (Fischman et al. 1986). There are discrepancies about the nature, pattern, magnitude and duration of these changes (Barclay et al. 1994). However, the interaction of pregnancy, childbirth, and sexual and marital relationships is poorly understood.

## Physiological changes during pregnancy

Physiological adjustments are necessary to provide an optimal environment for the developing fetus. This is a complex process that intimately involves all the systems in the body and begins from the moment of conception until after the birth of the baby. These physiological adaptations generally occur smoothly to minimize the effect of the normal function of the body (Chamberlain 1997). If women intend to exercise during pregnancy, the changes of pregnancy need to be carefully considered to ensure that a safe environment is always maintained for both mother and fetus.

### *Cardiovascular*

The purpose of the cardiovascular system is to provide oxygen and nutrients to the tissues of the body and to remove waste products of metabolism from the body. Cardiovascular changes during pregnancy are necessary to meet the extra demands for oxygen of the body tissues, which in turn need to meet the needs of the growing fetus and maternal organs as pregnancy progresses (Chamberlain 1997). Changes include a substantial increase in blood volume, which is compensated in part by increased venous capacity, cardiac dilatation and reduced peripheral vascular resistance (Wolfe et al. 1989a).

There is a physiological increase in blood volume of between 18% and 45% above the non-pregnant volume (Gorski 1985; de Swiet 1991a; Araujo 1997). This is mainly the result of an increase in plasma volume of up to 50% and a 20% increase in red blood cell volume. This leads to an overall dilution of these cells, and subsequently there are fewer red blood cells in a single area to transport oxygen than in a non-pregnant woman. The ability of the blood to carry oxygen is called the oxygen-carrying capacity and this results in the 'physiological anaemia of pregnancy' (de Swiet 1991a).

Relative to pre-pregnancy levels, cardiac output during rest increases gradually from between 30% and up to 50% starting at about week 8 of the first trimester of pregnancy, and reaches a maximum level at the beginning of the third trimester, becoming stable towards term. Resting heart rate increases by 15 beats/min (de Swiet 1991a; Duvekot et al. 1993, 1995; Araujo 1997). There is uncertainty about the exact timing and pattern of the component changes and the underlying factors responsible (de Swiet 1991a; Duvekot et al. 1995). Thus, the pregnant woman can never achieve a state at rest as she could before pregnancy or will achieve again after pregnancy.

The increase in circulating blood volume is not uniformly distributed throughout the body. Renal blood flow is increased during pregnancy by 40% and there is understandably a response to the increased demands of the uterine requirements (Chamberlain 1997). Other organ supplies such as hepatic and cerebral blood flow remain unchanged (Gorski 1985).

After the fourth month of pregnancy, the enlarging uterus is capable of interfering with venous return by compression of the inferior vena cava. This can cause supine hypertension syndrome, affecting cardiac output, and interfering with uterine circulation (Ueland et al. 1969; Sweet and Tiran 1997; Artal and Sherman 1999). To prevent this occurring, exercise should not be performed in the supine position after the first trimester of pregnancy.

The systemic vascular resistance is also markedly reduced as a result of both a reduction in vascular tone by high levels of progesterone and an increase in blood flow to the placenta and pregnant uterus (Schrier and Briner 1991). In early pregnancy, the relaxing effects of the hormone progesterone also lead to a decrease in blood pressure (Magness and Rosenfeld 1989; Omar et al. 1995). Systolic blood pressure remains relatively stable throughout pregnancy with a fall in diastolic blood pressure, being lowest at mid-pregnancy and then tends to reach non-pregnant values by term (Duvekot et al. 1993). In late pregnancy, blood pressure may even be too high as a result of a combination of hormonal influences and cardiovascular changes (Gorski 1985).

### Respiratory system

Extensive changes occur in the respiratory system where gas exchange takes place with the intake of oxygen and excretion of carbon dioxide. Changes include anatomical and functional alterations and are the result of hormonal influence, mainly progesterone. These changes occur before the growing uterus mechanically impairs ventilation.

In early pregnancy, women breathe more deeply but not more frequently under the influence of progesterone. The respiratory centre has increased sensitivity to carbon dioxide. Hence, minute ventilation increases by 50% above pre-pregnancy levels, which is far more than the need for gas exchange (Chamberlain 1991; Romen et al. 1991; de Swiet 1991b). The capacity for ventilation remains essentially normal throughout pregnancy. This is despite the progressive decrease in expiratory reserve volume and functional residual capacity in the second half of pregnancy (Pernoll et al. 1975; de Swiet 1991b).

Later the growing uterus increases intra-abdominal pressure so that the lower ribs flare out and the diaphragm is pushed upwards (Gorski 1985; Chamberlain 1991). In the third trimester, the bulky uterus can force the diaphragm up by as much as 4 cm, distorting the chest shape and size and resulting in a reduction in respiratory reserve. Anatomical changes in the respiratory system may cause women discomfort as pregnancy progresses.

### Endocrine factors

The placenta plays an important role as a multifunctional endocrine gland. The endocrine systems undergo profound changes during pregnancy, which are modulated by the ovaries, maternal endocrine glands and the placenta (Romen et al. 1991).

Pregnancy results in gestationally induced changes in plasma hormone levels of oestrogen, progesterone and relaxin. Oestrogen stimulates growth of the body tissues necessary to support the pregnancy. This includes growth and development of the uterus, placenta, fetus, breast tissue and extra muscle tissue within the heart. Progesterone has a relaxing effect on the smooth muscle within the body. This helps the cardiovascular system cope with the increasing demands of pregnancy. Other systems in the body, such as the digestive system, are also affected. The hormone relaxin is produced from the early weeks of pregnancy, reaches the highest level by the end of the first trimester and takes several months to return to normal after pregnancy. The main role of relaxin is to relax ligaments and connective tissues.

Pregnancy is a diabetogenic event especially through the action of the hormones cortisol, progesterone and human chorionic sommatomammotrophin. Hormone levels start to rise between 6 and 9 weeks and peak between 25 and 32 weeks of pregnancy. This predisposes to the body becoming more resistant to insulin in order to ensure that maternal blood glucose circulates within the system for longer periods (Sharp 1993). During pregnancy, fasting blood sugar and glucose levels tend to be lower than in the non-pregnant woman. As the pregnant woman uses carbohydrates at a greater rate during pregnancy, hypoglycaemia may occur under conditions of prolonged or strenuous exercise (Gorski 1985).

### Musculoskeletal system

Relaxin has the effect of softening the ligaments, making them more elastic and flexible (Dumas and Reid 1997). This affects mainly the pelvis–sacroiliac joints and pubic symphysis joint (Romen et al. 1991). From an obstetric point of view, this is desirable because it relaxes the ligaments of the pelvis and birth canal to accommodate the developing fetus and delivery of the baby. However, the hormones affect all joints, making them potentially unstable and putting them at risk of overstretching, especially in weight-bearing areas (Dumas and Reid 1997).

Spinal changes may be characterized by further development of lumbar lordosis. This is an exaggerated curvature in the lower back created to help bear the weight of the growing fetus towards term. Increased laxity of the pelvic and sacroiliac joints and loss of strength and tone of the abdominal muscles, as pregnancy progresses, may bring this about (Romen et al. 1991). As a result, the abdominal muscles become less efficient in their vital role of supporting the lower back and maintaining posture. Both lumbar lordosis and weaker abdominal muscles may cause additional strain on the back and can often create balance and coordination problems. Low back pain is a common recurrent complaint during pregnancy (Sharp 1993).

By 12 weeks of pregnancy, the enlarging uterus moves from the pelvic cavity to become an abdominal organ. The anterior orientation of the uterus expands into the abdominal cavity. This, along with changes in the breast, displaces the woman's centre of gravity upwards and forwards, resulting in rotation of the pelvis on the femur. A change in the centre of gravity puts extra work on the muscles to keep the body 'in balance'. It can make the body unstable, either at rest or for any kind of movement, resulting in the woman 'relearning' how to stand or to move (McNitt-Gray 1991; Sharp 1993).

Other problems of particular concern at this time include nerve compression syndromes and more rarely separation of the symphysis pubis. In the third trimester, the pregnant woman commonly experiences reduced mobility of ankle joints and wrists in spite of increased relaxation of the ligaments. Fluid retention, mainly in the ground substance of the connective tissue, causes these changes. This results in marked visible ankle oedema and paraesthesia in the hands, muscular weakness, and the carpal and tarsal tunnel syndromes (Tobin 1967).

### Oxygen consumption

The progressive increases in cardiac output and pulmonary ventilation are proportionally greater than those occurring in maternal and fetal consumption during pregnancy (de Swiet 1991b). The resting oxygen intake rises significantly from around 18 weeks to between 15% and 20% above normal during pregnancy (Gorski 1985; de Swiet 1991b). The initial increase is primarily caused by increased cardiac and renal energy costs. The major increase in resting oxygen consumption occurs during the second half of pregnancy and is the result of the rapidly growing fetus and the enlarging placenta and uterus (de Swiet 1991b).

### Nutritional and energy requirements

The estimated energy cost of pregnancy is approximately 80 000 kilocalories (kcal) in total or 300 kcal/day. These required extra kilocalories meet the metabolic needs of pregnancy and the developing fetus. The energy demand is unevenly distributed, with most energy being required in the middle 20 weeks of pregnancy mainly as a result of fat storage during this period. Thus, the demands are less at the beginning and end of the pregnancy when fat storage does not occur. This energy cost of pregnancy can be met either by increasing calorie intake or by reducing energy expenditure (King et al. 1994).

A healthy average woman during the course of her pregnancy can gain between 11 and 13 kg in weight, depending on maternal diet, activity levels and other factors pertaining to gestation, such as 'morning sickness' and multiple pregnancies. The growing fetus, placenta, amniotic fluids and increase in circulating body fluids, breast and other body tissues, and body fat contribute to this overall weight gain (Sweet and Tiran 1997).

# Exercise and the healthy individual

Exercise is an important instrument in health promotion to encourage individuals to change behaviour and develop lifelong skills for exercise (Patrick et al. 1994). Individuals tend to view exercise from either a negative or a positive perspective. In general, most forms of exercise are associated with positive aspects of physical fitness which signifies a sense of 'well-being'.

Physical activity is closely related to, but distinct from, exercise and physical fitness. Physical activity has been defined as any bodily movement produced by skeletal muscles that result in energy expenditure (Caspersen et al. 1985). Exercise is a subset of physical activity and has been defined as 'planned, structured and repetitive bodily movements done to improve or maintain one or more components of physical fitness'. Physical fitness is a set of attributes that people have or achieve which relates to the ability to perform physical activity (Caspersen et al. 1985).

Exercise physiology is concerned with the functional changes within the body brought about by participation in acute or chronic exposure to physical exercise often with improvement in the physiological response to exercise. Acute exercise is a physiological stressor, which requires a major haemostatic adjustment in all major organs. The common difference in the physiological response to chronic exercise among individuals depends on several factors, including age, body weight and body composition, the muscles involved, physical condition, nutritional status, motivation, body position, exercise regime and the environment in which the activity is undertaken.

Aerobic exercise requires metabolic processes that use oxygen from inspired air, which is delivered to exercising muscles by the cardiovascular system. It involves large muscle groups working in a steady rhythm; such exercises include walking, running and cycling. Anaerobic exercise uses processes that do not primarily use oxygen from inspired air, and are explosive-type exercises of short duration such as weight lifting (Lamb 1984).

Observations suggest that a complex interaction of many variables will determine individual attitudes and behaviour towards exercise. Consideration should be given to underlying motives for exercising besides the common and fully conscious reason to 'feel better' (Allied Dunbar National Fitness Survey [ADNFS] 1992).

## Physical and health benefits of exercise

Regular physical activity has long been regarded as an important component of a healthy lifestyle (Pate et al. 1995). There is general agreement that exercise performed by healthy individuals of all ages has both physical and psychological benefits. These include improved psychological well-being, physical performance and enhanced quality of life (Bouchard et al. 1994). Some of the most important physical benefits supported by a wealth of scientific evidence include increased stamina and reserve to cope with extra physical demands, maintenance of muscle strength, tone and joint flexibility, and management of body weight (ADNFS 1992).

There is a belief that regular physical activity, resulting in physical fitness, has health benefits for individuals as well as the implications for medical care of individuals with certain medical conditions and diseases (Bouchard et al. 1994). These include a reduced risk of coronary heart disease, better control of blood pressure in cases of mild hypertension, prevention of osteoporosis, management of hyperlipidaema and glycaemic control, improved weight control and alleviation of disabilities (ADNFS 1992; Bouchard et al. 1994). It is interesting to note that findings have emerged to challenge the assumption that cardiovascular benefits are similar for males and females (Douglas 1994; Wenger 1998). This may be incorrect as a result of the physiological differences between the sexes and further research is now required in women.

There have been suggestions that exercise may affect longevity or that a reversal of ageing may occur. A number of epidemiological studies have attempted to examine the long-term effects of exercise on longevity. Exercise programmes for those aged over 65 years of both sexes are strongly associated with the maintenance of functional ability and maintenance of independence (Fiatarone et al. 1994; Posner et al. 1995). There is well-documented evidence of the benefit of exercise training in relation to the normal age-related decline in peak performance and maximal aerobic capacity, loss of muscle, bone mass, increase in body fat and modification or retardation of the ageing process.

The beneficial effects of exercise are likely to involve many factors. Exercise is associated with lower body weight, a lower percentage of body fat, lower incidence of cigarette smoking, lower blood pressure and lower total cholesterol levels (Gibbons et al. 1983). Exercise affects the incidence of coronary heart disease by reducing the risk factors for the development of the disease, although the mechanism for this effect remains unclear (Morris et al. 1980; Berlin and Colditz 1990; Morris 1995).

Chronic adaptations in physiological function, developed as a result of physical training, are generally believed to have benefits to the individual to such an extent that it may influence mortality and morbidity (Gibbons et al. 1983; Blair et al. 1989). Despite well-documented evidence of the benefits of exercise, there are detrimental effects such as cardiovascular accidents (CVAs) and sudden death when exercise is undertaken by an unsuitable participant or carried out in an inappropriate environment.

### Specific health benefits for women

Anecdotal evidence suggests that physical activity is particularly beneficial to women (Harris 1981; Berger 1984; Tanji 2000). A recent review of empirical evidence supports the promotion of exercise to improve physical and mental health in women (Choi and Mutrie 1996). In particular, recent reviews have suggested that physical activity may enhance bone density and this could help protect women against osteoporosis (Gannon 1988; Marcus et al. 1992). Osteoporosis is the medical term for a condition in which there is a decrease in bone density, rendering the skeleton susceptible to fractures. Women are more at risk of this condition than men as a result of the acceleration of bone loss caused by cessation of ovarian function during and after the menopause. Findings from clinical trials suggest that appropriate weight-bearing activity may enhance bone density by 4%, which is similar to the improvements noted from drug therapies (Simkin et al. 1987; Smith et al. 1990).

Regular exercise may benefit the alleviation of the symptoms associated with the menstrual cycle. This includes improvements in levels of low back and pelvic pain, headaches, anxiety, depression and fatigue. Over-training or regular participation in vigorous exercise may also have potential adverse effects on menstrual function and eating disorders (Tanji 2000). However, experts in this area believe that the benefits outweigh the risks associated with menstrual function (Lebrun 1994).

There remains uncertainty as to whether regular exercise can reduce the risk of cancer because of inconclusive findings and other confounding variables. Women who were physically active were found to have a reduction in the risk of breast cancer (Thune et al. 1997) and cancer of the reproductive organs (Frisch et al. 1987). Other studies did not find any association between exercise and reduced risk of breast cancer (Rockhill et al. 1998). Further studies are required to confirm a causal relationship between exercise and a decrease in the rate of breast cancer (Tanji 2000).

Health promotion and disease prevention are of prime importance in reducing mortality and morbidity rates. The focus of health enhancement through physical activity is now widely proposed and achieving health through exercise and fitness has been central to many contemporary health promotion programmes (Fahlberg and Fahlberg 1996). An increasingly active society is likely to have a major impact in reducing the economic and social costs caused by chronic ill-health or premature death, and could improve the quality of life for millions of people (ADNFS 1992).

## Psychological benefits of exercise

Exercise contributes to achieving optimal psychological health (ADNFS 1992). Numerous affective benefits are associated with both acute and chronic physical activity (Brown and Harrison 1986; Roth and Holmes 1987). The physiological basis for these effects remains unclear.

Over the last 20 years, research has demonstrated the positive effects and associations between physical activity and psychological well-being in both normal and clinical populations. These include positive mood, decreased levels of anxiety and depression (McCann and Holmes 1984), enhanced self-esteem (Hughes 1984) and increased ability to cope with stress (Brown and Harrison 1986; Crews and Landers 1987; Stephens 1988; ADNFS 1992). A meta-analysis of studies in these areas suggests that exercise either acts as a coping strategy or serves as an 'inoculator' to enable individuals to respond more effectively to psychosocial stress; exercise thus provides an efficient coping system for stress (Crews and Landers 1987).

Physical activity has been found to be positively associated with general well-being, lower levels of anxiety and depression, and more positive mood (Stephens 1988; Crammer et al. 1991). Women have reported an improvement in coping abilities and reduced tension/anxiety levels after following a moderate exercise programme (Morgan 1979, 1985; Moses et al. 1989; Steptoe et al. 1989). Other reported benefits of exercise programmes for the normal population include: enhancement of mood (Roth and Holmes 1987; North et al. 1990), improved self-confidence, feelings of achievement and self-satisfaction and self-sufficiency (Brown and Harrison 1986).

Physical activity may help people to cope more effectively and reduce emotional reaction to stressful life events (Steptoe 1992). Steptoe et al. (1989) concluded that moderate exercise in inactive adults led to significant improvements in aerobic fitness and was associated with significantly greater reductions in tension, anxiety and depression with increases in the perceived ability to cope with stress. Loughlan (1995) found that sedentary employees who had increased their physical activity levels could significantly improve coping deficits and contribute to improvements in coping abilities.

Self-concept is the picture that individuals have of 'their own self' and is formed by the perceptions that they have of their physical domain, including physical capacities and awareness of body image and attractiveness (Fox 1988; Fox and Corbin 1989). Self-esteem is a personal judgement of one's own overall worth (Fox 1988).

In general, individuals who exercise tend to report more positive subjective indicators of psychological well-being than non-exercising counterparts. Findings from research studies indicate that exercise is associated with improvements in mental health. Researchers speculate that self-esteem and self-control are mediating factors that increase with exercise (Tanji 2000). These factors may explain the beneficial effect of exercise on mood and mental health. Many factors may be involved in this association, but a single causal link has not yet been established (Raglin 1990; Thirlaway and Benton 1996).

It can be concluded that women who exercise regularly are likely to be more comfortable with day-to-day physical exertion and have reduced anxiety and improved body image. It is generally thought that physical activity leads to an improved quality of life (ADNFS 1992) despite subjective indicators of psychological well-being being difficult to measure. Individuals who are regularly active may be more likely to adopt other 'health lifestyle' behaviours (Jamieson and Flood 1993).

### Mechanisms proposed for psychological benefits

Most authorities currently agree that exercise reduces tension and improves mental health. However, a specific 'cause and effect' has not been identified and uncertainty remains about the mechanisms that can be attributed to the psychological benefits experienced by those who exercise.

The 'endorphin hypothesis' was first proposed in the 1970s and remains a popular hypothesis to explain affective benefits associated with exercise. This hypothesis focuses on the knowledge that the brain, pituitary gland and other tissues produce various endorphins. Their subsequent action with exercise could be 'morphine like', in the sense that they have the ability to reduce the sense of pain and produce a state of euphoria or the much-publicized 'exercise high' (Morgan 1985). However, it is unlikely that this hypothesis alone could provide the answer to all the complex neurobiological factors involved in mood alterations associated with exercise.

La Forge (1995) undertook a comprehensive review of the literature related to the most popular hypothetical neurobiological mechanisms that underpin exercise-related mood alterations. Nearly all hypotheses were recognized to overlap or share some common neuroanatomical pathway. The most likely explanation for exercise-induced affective changes was concluded to evolve from an integration of brain neuro-transmission processes involving the principal neuroactive substances, such as noradrenaline (norepinephrine or NA), serotonin (5-hydroxy-tryptamine or 5HT), endorphin, dopamine and enkephalin. La Forge suggested that the probable mechanism responsible for mood change was the extraordinary influences of biological transactions, including genetic, environmental, and acute and adaptive neurobiological processes. The final answers are likely to emerge in the future as a result of the combined action of researchers and theorists from exercise science, cognitive science and neurobiology.

# Historical overview of exercise in obstetrics

Attitudes to child-bearing and physical activity have emerged and changed over the centuries and have varied considerably from culture to culture and generation to generation. A possible interrelationship of maternal physical activity, pregnancy and birth outcome has been recognized throughout history since biblical times. Hard-working Hebrew women tended to have easier and shorter labours than Egyptian women who led an indolent and sedentary lifestyle (Exodus I, 19).

### Fifteenth to eighteenth centuries

During the Tudor and Stuart times in England, obstetricians made similar observations with women from different social backgrounds. Although childbirth for rich and respectable women was believed to be painful and dangerous, it was not thought to be so for those women from lower social orders (Eccles 1982).

> Sometimes the hardy Scots or the wild Irish were said to have almost painless labours and sometimes working country women.
>
> Eccles (1982, p. 86)

One may speculate that this could be associated with the very different quality of lifestyle experienced by women from different social classes. Hard-working women from lower classes may have experienced easier and shorter labours as a result of delivering relatively small infants and the predisposition to pre-term or precipitous labours. Conversely, indolent and sedentary women from higher classes may have delivered much larger infants resulting in longer labour and possibly associated dystocia.

The belief that rich and sedentary women had more difficult labours, compared with those of poor hard-worked women, acquired a social cachet (Eccles 1982). This was desirable for physicians because it was essential that they attended 'women of quality' assiduously during confinement. Undoubtedly, this would be beneficial 'to increase their own importance, and hence their fees' (Eccles 1982, p. 90). Physicians had deemed themselves the rightful experts about all aspects of women, their health and lifestyle. This had an important long-lasting legacy on the outlook of middle-class women and how they should behave and live their lives.

The philosophy during the seventeenth and eighteenth centuries was to encourage women to exercise during pregnancy, albeit within the lifestyle and social limitations of this period (Harvey 1950; Eccles 1982; Gelis 1991). English writers acknowledged advice in relation to physical activity to ensure good health during pregnancy and to prevent miscarriage. Pregnant women were advised to take a sedan or a litter as opposed to riding horseback or in a coach, and to avoid dressing their own hair to prevent straining the ligaments of the womb upwards. The best sort of exercise to undertake was walking in low-heeled shoes and they could continue to exercise the arms by spinning or carding (Eccles 1982).

Barrett (1699) claimed that the correct ordering of the classic non-naturals – air, food, drink, exercise and rest, sleep and waking, fullness and emptiness, and passion of the mind – would keep pregnant women in good frame for childbirth, unlike the fine ladies who pampered themselves (cited in Eccles 1982, p. 61). A universal fear was the possibility of strangling the infant with the umbilical cord. As a precaution, pregnant women were advised to avoid any activity that involved circular movements such as unwinding skeins of wool or grinding coffee (Gelis 1991).

During the seventeenth century, many obstetricians advised women to increase the amount of exercise close to the time of delivery, whereas others disagreed with this advice. Mauriceau (1683) strongly believed that exercise could predispose to the child turning sideways or into some other malposition and result in hard labour (cited in Eccles 1982):

> . . . instead of giving herself rest, she falls a jumping, walking, running up and down stairs and so forth, the child would very likely turn sideways or in some other wrong position.
>
> Eccles (1982, pp. 61–2)

Louise Bourgeois, a renowned French midwife, who was one of the first women to write in obstetrics, had a similar view of exercise. She believed that exercise in the late stages of pregnancy would dilate the belly, drag down the womb and bruise the child's head against the mother's pelvis (Harvey 1950, p. 215).

Eighteenth-century doctors were free with advice and criticism and were interested in the regulation in lifestyle of pregnant women (Gelis 1991). Alexander Hamilton was Professor of Midwifery at the University of Edinburgh, who published the first edition of his *Treatise of Midwifery* in 1781. In this he gave 'Rules and Caution for the Conduct of Pregnant Women' which included the following recommendations:

> Women when pregnant should lead a regular and temperate life carefully avoiding whatever is observed to disagree with the stomach; . . . their exercise should be moderate, and adapted to their particular situation; they should, especially in the early months when the connection between ovum and womb is feeble, avoid crowds, confinement, every situation which renders them under any disagreeable restriction; agitation of body from violent or improper exercise, as jolting in a carriage, riding on horseback, dancing and whatever disturbs either body or mind.
>
> Munro Kerr et al. (1954, p. 145)

In a paper read to the Medical Society of London in 1788, James Lucas, a surgeon at Leeds General Infirmary, advocated 'an increase in exercise' during pregnancy. He suggested that exercise would reduce the size of the child and may help overcome difficulty in labour in the event of a woman having a contracted pelvis (Munro Kerr et al. 1954, p.145).

In France, it was customary for women to remain inactive during early pregnancy when the fetus's hold on life was fragile. However, physicians opposed continued inactivity throughout pregnancy because they believed that exercise was necessary to nourish good health of the pregnant woman. They advised that walking was by far the best exercise for pregnant women while it was necessary 'to refrain from extremes either too much or too little' in relation to dancing jigs and reels (Gelis 1991, p. 78).

### Nineteenth century

Some obstetricians realized the importance of exercise in the antenatal period. Thomas Bull (1837), in one of the first books solely devoted to antenatal care, advised that physical activity and the need for outdoor air were prerequisites for a healthy pregnancy (cited in Munro Kerr et al. 1954). He cautioned against all agitating exercises and, in short, really said do not run, do not jump, do not drive unsafe horses, give up dancing and riding, and do not plunge in cold water. Moderate gentle daily exercise in the open air was preferred if possible and should always include a share of housework (Smith 1979).

The nineteenth century was also a period of paradox in terms of women and their bodies. This era in Britain was dominated by offensive and patronizing attitudes towards pregnancy, which were initiated and perpetuated by a patriarchal society. The Victorian doctor influenced women to view their bodies and natural functions in a discerning way. American society also encouraged compliance of women, which was instilled from childhood (Donnelly 1988).

Social etiquette during the Victorian age in England was deemed to be of prime importance for middle- and upper-class women. Women of this status strove for the ideal status symbol of 'true womanhood' represented in the passive, weak, frail and delicate female. This indolent, inactive lifestyle was in contrast to that of lower-class women who relied on their bodies for survival and who viewed physical strength and endurance as a valued commodity for survival (Lutter 1994).

The pregnant well-bred lady of this era had to be reticent and was advised to rest and undertake the minimal physical activity possible. Attitudes towards physical capabilities of women had an impact on the lifestyle and outlook of middle-class women. They avoided social company during pregnancy because of the adverse effect that they might create in others in society (Blankfield 1967). Most early women doctors continued to promote the very notions of Victorian delicacy and decorum so strongly endorsed by their male counterparts. This contributed to keeping women enclosed in their separate sphere in society.

Many women did challenge traditional roles and behavioural prescriptions at this time. During the second half of the nineteenth century, the growing history of participation in exercise was testimony to the fact that more women were not paying any attention to the medical cautions about overuse and overstrain in exercise. Many women viewed exercise as a release from some of the more entrenched and pervasive tenets of the Victorian ideology of femininity (McCrone 1988).

Orthodox doctors were generally committed to forbidding exercise during and after pregnancy. Women had to rest horizontally after child-birth to guard against ligament stain and prolapse of the womb (Pancoast 1859, cited in Vertinsky 1990). This was 3–4 days and much longer for delicate women. Too many labours were probably the reason for frequent prolapse of the womb but, despite this, the argument that too much vigorous exercise might strain ligaments of the uterus has been invoked many times to restrain women in physical activity and sport (Smith 1979).

Pregnancy was regarded as needing special exercise, close medical advice and supervision. The expectant woman had to conserve her resources, because she was living for two and the child's future depended on the mother's conduct during pregnancy (Holbrook 1875). From the beginning of pregnancy, more care than usual should be taken to use regular, abundant and helpful exercise. Holbrook advised that exercise in the morning would be more beneficial to secure the two advantages of using the best physical strength, thus avoiding additional risk from exertion when the body is fatigued and the best use of sunshine and air. Walking in the open air within limitations was consistently promoted as the most suitable activity for pregnant women (Green 1892; Galabin 1900). There was now no question that most women would benefit from such exercise and consequently have easier labours (Green 1892).

Physicians agreed that the amount of exercise was to be determined by the needs of the female body at each stage of the reproductive devel-opment. The craze of bicycle riding emerging in the 1890s had a revolutionary role in expanding women's views of physical mobility that often stimulated contradictory advice from physicians. The estab-lished medical journals increasingly portrayed the pros and cons of bicycling upon female health during that decade, and women needed to consult their physician before riding a bicycle.

Bicycling used by women with direction and sense was thought to encourage strengthening abdominal muscle, more stable nerves, easier labours and healthy children (Pendergast 1896). More specifically, some believed that bicycling would strengthen the muscles of the uterus to make childbirth easier. This was in contrast to horse-riding which was believed to produce a funnel-shaped pelvis and posed diffi-culties for child-bearing (Garrigus 1896, cited in Vertinsky 1990). It was further argued that strengthening the leg muscles would stimulate pelvic tone, strengthening the pelvis and restoring reproductive normalcy (Dickinson 1895). Vigorous debates arose as to whether overuse of the bicycle resulted in acute and chronic conditions in those areas previously suggested to have benefits: jarring and jolting may cause uterine displacement and spinal shock, and pelvic organ damage and overstretching and hardening of the abdominal muscles were especially targeted for possible problems in labour (Fenton 1896, cited in Vertinsky 1990).

Other physical and sporting activities were increasingly being accepted by establishment positions to strengthen women for child-birth and as a tonic to revive their enthusiasm for their housewifely duties. These included riding, hunting, tennis, rowing and golf. Rowing was thought to harden the muscles, strengthen the back and increase the breathing power of the lungs.

Late nineteenth-century physicians were among the first of the new experts to claim a scientific foundation for their medical pronounce-ments on how women should look and behave, and what they were capable of doing physically. An interaction of social perception, medical practice and scientific knowledge influenced views about the amount and type of physical activity taken by women during pregnancy. An interrelationship of physical activity, social class and the birthweight of infants was recognized and acknowledged during the nineteenth century. Published scientific studies demonstrated that women from lower social classes gave birth to lighter babies than their counterparts from higher social classes (Pinard 1885, cited in Artal Mittlemark and Gardin 1991, page 2). Letourner (1886) concluded that strong 'robust' women engaged in strenuous physical work deliv-ered lower-birthweight babies than lighter women involved in less demanding work (cited in Artal Mittlemark and Gardin 1991, p. 2).

Ballantyne (1903) also advocated that antenatal exercises and training in relaxation techniques would benefit pregnant women during their labour (cited in Munro Kerr et al. 1954, p. 146). The concept that women of lower social classes had far easier labours compared with their rich counterparts was attributed to differences in levels of physical activity (Munro Kerr et al. 1954). This idea was developed to such an extent that uterine inertia was subsequently attributed to lack of exercise (Haultain and Fahmy 1929).

On these grounds, advice was often full of admonitions and warnings. Walking outdoors and gentle exercise were regarded as necessary in pregnancy and women were advised that difficult labours were likely if they avoided these activities. In contrast, stooping, lifting, and any violent and sudden forms of activity were deemed particularly harmful to pregnancy and could induce miscarriage (Munro Kerr et al. 1954). Pregnant women were recommended to walk outdoors in moderation and partake in gentle forms of exercises which included croquet, bathing, swimming, golf and ballroom dancing. They were also advised to avoid horse riding, and violent and sudden forms of activity that were deemed particularly harmful to pregnancy (Munro Kerr et al. 1954).

Historians caution that there was a diversity of opinions and issues about twentieth-century attitudes towards the nature and place of women, and to be meaningful these controversies must be placed carefully in their social and cultural context. Women even within the same social class did not have the same experiences and were not uniformly oppressed. Literature on guidance for health and exercise behaviour was readily available, although inflexible for middle-class women only. However, literature did extend substantially for working-class women during the first two decades of the twentieth century (McCrone 1988).

## Twentieth century (1900–1960)

During the first few decades of the twentieth century, Fairbairn (1926) advocated that 'natural childbirth' could be achieved through antenatal and relaxation exercises and he termed this 'constructive physiology' (Montgomery 1969). He was the first to propose that some form of physical preparation could benefit women during pregnancy to prepare for childbirth. This 'preventative outlook' for childbirth was one of the most progressive features of obstetrics during this era (Munro Kerr et al. 1954). Fairbairn believed that prenatal exercise and relaxation contributed to women gaining confidence to cope with the stress of labour. Specialized exercise programmes to prepare women for childbirth were first introduced during the late 1920s and early 1930s, and Fairbairn included prenatal instruction as part of the scope of his unit at St Thomas' Hospital, London (Montgomery 1969).

Many doctors and midwives found that education with certain physical exercises and training in relaxation before childbirth proved to be beneficial during and after childbirth. It was now generally believed that women could be physically prepared to undertake the muscular feat of labour, which may possibly be the greatest feat that many women would ever undertake. Dick-Read (1933), Randall (1939) and Morris (1936) were English pioneers in the field of antenatal education who were influenced by this concept and advocated antenatal preparation for childbirth. The importance of the psychological benefits gained by exercise was subsequently recognized within contemporary programmes (Munro Kerr et al. 1954).

During the 1930s, Dick-Read developed and introduced specific breathing and exercises to prepare women physically for labour. He popularized the theory that fear leads to tension, which in turn causes pain in childbirth. He believed that labour was not necessarily an inherently painful process and the pain experienced by women during labour arose from socially induced expectations about pain. The physically-based programme aimed to improve health, muscle tone and a 'sense of well-being', in addition to building up confidence and reducing the pain of childbirth (Dick-Read 1933). Initially, Dick-Read's teachings were practised and more widely accepted abroad, particularly in the USA, than in Britain (Munro Kerr et al. 1954, p. 156).

Morris (1936) and Randall (1939) were largely responsible for the development of antenatal and postnatal exercise programmes. Morris (1936) in collaboration with Randall devised an exercise programme to enhance therapeutic benefits of exercise during and after pregnancy. This programme aimed to enhance physical and mental well-being through adaptation of controlled movements to the specific needs of pregnant women and mothers. Benefits included improved posture, muscle tone, strengthening pelvic and abdominal muscles, and psychological preparation for motherhood. The most beneficial was found to be the positive mental attitude adopted by new mothers on the programme. The use of exercise during and after pregnancy was not new, but the value of exercise had not been fully appreciated until this time.

Kathleen Vaughan was an obstetrician whose influence was felt in the same unit as Fairbairn. She found that women who led an active life in the open air had their babies easier than those women from Kashmir who lived in purdah with its strict rules on seclusion, had very little exercise or sunlight and delivered their babies with difficulty. She maintained that the more confined and artificial way of life resulted in greater complications of child-bearing. As a result, she initiated exercise classes in London with the aim of helping town-bred civilized women to have their babies naturally and easily. Vaughan (1942) held the view that flexible joints were an essential factor for an easy labour, in addition to a well-developed and normally shaped pelvis and an unconstrained attitude for delivery. She believed that women should adopt a squatting position or exaggerated lithotomy position during labour, to encourage the pelvic joints to open out and allow an easier passage for delivery of the baby through the birth canal. Women were encouraged to adopt tailor-sitting positions and also to perform pelvic floor exercises to increase the elasticity and tonicity of the perineum and prevent perineal trauma. These practices continued despite being subsequently proven not to enlarge the pelvis and also to be a potential source of injury to women (Young 1940).

Randall (1939) recommended squatting and lunging exercises during pregnancy to widen the pubic arch and shorten the anterior wall of the birth canal to aid the delivery process. Vaughan (1951) suggested that women who exercised regularly were likely to have an easier confinement than sedentary woman. She associated a sedentary lifestyle with difficulty in childbirth as a result of stunted growth and development of the pelvis. She also advocated that all women should undertake specialized exercise programmes in a group situation as part of their physical preparation for labour and delivery (cited in Munro Kerr et al. 1954):

> The mother who has lived a natural life from her own birth, who was breastfed herself and who has lived on plain, good food, with plenty of free movement in the fresh air when growing, she is the woman who will have an easy confinement when her time comes; while the more luxurious, wrapped-up bottlefed infant, kept long hours in a perambulator or indoors, with no exercise, and later sitting long hours in school, is very likely to have difficulty in childbearing later on because the natural growth, shape and mobility of the pelvis and its joints have been stunted.

Lamaze was another pioneer of modern childbirth preparation who introduced the psychoprophylactic method of painless childbirth to the Western World during the 1950s. This 'Lamaze method' did not place any direct emphasis on exercise to prepare women psychologically, but did include exercises within the programme to prepare women physically for childbirth (Lamaze 1958). The Russian, Nicolaiev, initially coined psychoprophylaxis in 1949 to classify a system claimed to originate in his homeland. He explained and demonstrated the method at a medical conference in Leningrad in 1951, with two colleagues, Velvosky and Platonov. Briefly there are two elements involved in psychoprophylaxis, with the first one based on Pavlov's theory of conditioned reflexes that says that from childhood we associate pain with childbirth. This is not an inborn attribute of women and these pernicious associations can be replaced by beneficial associations through reconditioning. Pain would not be a problem if these were maintained through education, building up confidence and continued support. The second element is based on a focus of activity to raise the pain threshold. It is suggested that a programme of physical and mental activity, demanding a focus of attention and concentration, can block the painful stimuli of labour from reaching the part of the brain that becomes conscious, resulting in the need for less pain relief.

Heardman (1959) advocated that physical training for childbirth promoted good health, poise, good posture and good body mechanics during and after pregnancy. She had previously recommended the use of pelvic tilting and rocking during pregnancy and labour because these were considered to be invaluable exercises in the relief of low back strain (Heardman 1951).

The importance of antenatal education and exercise in relation to the psychological and physical preparation of women for labour and childbirth was now widely accepted by obstetricians. This acceptance resulted in the initiation of antenatal classes, which were established on a large scale. The content of the classes mainly included relaxation and breathing exercises with some gentle physical exercise to tone limbs and strengthen abdominal muscles (Munro Kerr et al. 1954). Advice pertaining to exercise was a common feature offered during antenatal care (Stern and Burnett 1958, p. 48):

> Outdoor exercise equivalent to walking one mile should be taken each day regularly during pregnancy. Violent sudden forms of exercise and lifting heavy weights should be avoided, as well as any straining or arduous domestic work. Horse riding is considered particularly harmful.

In one of the first research studies to investigate the value of antenatal exercise programmes in relation to pregnancy and birth outcome, Burnett (1956) reported that little benefit was gained from either physical or psychological preparation for childbirth. He recommended that attendants should forge cooperative relationships with individual women as opposed to large group sessions. Recommendations and contraindications for exercise were a common feature offered during antenatal care (Stern and Burnett 1958).

Anecdotal information gained over the centuries about the association between exercise and childbirth is now supported by scientific evidence. In general, there is a belief in the value of safe exercise for the healthy pregnant woman, provided that advice is appropriate to individual needs (Huch and Erkkola 1990; Artal and Sherman 1999).

Modern-day midwifery practice adopts a holistic approach to care by recognizing individual needs of women during and after pregnancy. Therefore, antenatal and postnatal exercise programmes do remain an important component for those women wanting to continue with an active lifestyle during and after childbirth. Although exercise programmes are not a prerequisite for all women during pregnancy and childbirth, they may contribute to the preparation of women to meet the physical and emotional challenges presented by pregnancy and the transition to parenthood.

# Scientific investigations of exercise during pregnancy

The response to exercise is determined by a number of psychological and physiological factors. Regular physical activity has become an integral part of life for many women and the fundamental concern is to what extent responses to exercise during pregnancy differ from those in the non-pregnant state.

Over the last 30 years, a wealth of research evidence has emerged in terms of the physiological response to exercise during pregnancy. Scientific advances in technology have allowed sophisticated assessment of maternal and fetal responses to exercise conditions. However, to date, the most reliable physiological data are derived from animal studies, which continue to be of great value in understanding the physiology and regulation of pregnancy, and the biology of the interaction between pregnancy and exercise.

It is important to recognize the strengths and limitations of the various animal models of obtaining information with potential human relevance. The strength of animal models lies in the experimental design, which allows control over multiple confounding factors, as well as the ability to control and measure directly the independent and dependent variables associated with an intervention. Animal studies allow a more invasive approach from which correlations in structure and function can readily be obtained. However, important differences in animal physiology and behaviour suggest that results of such studies may be of limited application to humans. It has been necessary to consider the physiological findings from animal studies because associated ethical and legal problems prohibit similar studies being performed on humans.

A review of scientific investigations over the last 30 years is presented in this section of the literature review. Early and recent research evidence and anecdotal information relevant to the physiological, physical and psychological effects of exercise during pregnancy are discussed. The subsections include: maternal physiological considerations; fetal physiological considerations; clinical outcomes in relation to pregnancy and birth outcomes; maternal musculoskeletal considerations; and psychological benefits. A brief summary of the main findings is presented at the end of each subsection and the areas of interest associated with the present study are reviewed in more detail.

The gaps in the literature are highlighted and those gaps to be addressed within the present study identified. The aims of the present study are detailed. There is also clarification of some of the terminology used within the review, in addition to the glossary of terms previously provided. This is intended to help the reader who may be new to research within the area of exercise and pregnancy.

## Maternal physiological considerations

Pregnancy is known to have a major impact on the circulatory system. There is concern that significant cardiovascular changes induced by exercise may have potential adverse effects on the fetus as a result of the selective redistribution of blood flow to the working muscles away from the splanchnic organs. In the normal healthy pregnant woman, such occurrences should be rarely encountered during mild and moderate exercise, but are more likely to occur during strenuous and prolonged exercise (Artal Mittlemark et al. 1991a).

In earlier studies in this area, researchers concluded that the increase in cardiac output with light or moderate exercise during pregnancy was well within normal limits for non-pregnant women Ueland et al. (1969) and similar to levels after pregnancy (Guzman and Caplan 1970). More recently, Pivarnik et al. (1993) found that physically fit women who continued to exercise during pregnancy had an enhanced and maintained cardiopulmonary response to exercise compared with sedentary women. Pivarnik et al. (1994) also reported that physically active women had significantly greater vascular volumes than their sedentary counterparts, which were maintained throughout pregnancy with continued exercise.

The individual's capacity for exercise is limited by the combined ability of the cardiovascular and respiratory systems to meet the increased demands of the muscles. During pregnancy, oxygen consumption measured at rest increases with advancing gestation to a maximum level of between 15% and 20% above the normal level at term (Lotgering et al. 1985). The major increase in resting oxygen consumption occurs during the second half of pregnancy and is a result of the rapidly growing fetus, enlarging placenta and uterus (Hytten and Chamberlain 1991).

Many women, especially those who are involved in competitive or endurance activities, are keen to continue exercising throughout pregnancy. There is now growing concern that the pressures to exercise and the competitive spirit that challenges some women may result in some placing performance goals above safety by striving to improve or maintain training levels (Hale and Artal Mittlemark 1991). Therefore, scientific research has focused on the extent to which exercise undertaken during pregnancy can improve physical fitness and elicit a training effect.

One of the best measures of physical fitness is the non-invasive measurement of maximal oxygen consumption ($VO_{2max}$) which is a measure of cardiovascular endurance. This includes a circulatory component to oxygen uptake (oxygen delivery) and an extraction component (oxygen utilization). Maximal oxygen consumption ($VO_{2max}$) is defined as the maximal rate at which oxygen can be used by the cells in the body (Lamb 1984). The evaluation of 'functional aerobic capacity' best describes the individual's capacity to meet and sustain daily weight-bearing activities whereas 'absolute aerobic capacity' is a measure of the individual's maximal cardiopulmonary capacity and maximal energy output by aerobic processes. In many instances, it is not advisable for subjects to perform at maximal exercise and therefore submaximal exercise tests give some indication of exercise tolerance.

Reports from the early literature are varied in relation to aerobic capacity or oxygen consumption. Findings suggest that aerobic capacity or oxygen consumption may be unaffected by exercise during pregnancy (Guzman and Caplan 1970), or increased during pregnancy (Collings et al. 1983) but does not remain elevated after delivery (Knuttgen and Emerson 1974; Pernoll et al. 1975). Recent findings support some earlier studies in relation to the increase in aerobic capacity or oxygen consumption during pregnancy, but suggest that levels also continue to remain elevated in the postpartum period (Clapp and Capeless 1991; Pivarnik et al. 1991). These reported studies are based on varying methodologies and some recent studies are given in more detail.

Pivarnik et al. (1991) found that oxygen consumption was higher from the start of the third trimester of pregnancy and remained elevated after delivery in previously sedentary women ($n = 16$) who exercised during pregnancy from 13 weeks' gestation onwards. Women exercised on the bicycle ergometer and treadmill and testing was carried out at 4-weekly intervals until 3 months postpartum. Functional aerobic capacity ($VO_2$ in ml/kg per min) during treadmill exercise was unchanged throughout pregnancy and the postpartum period. Absolute aerobic capacity ($VO_2$ in ml/min) was found to increase from 25 weeks' gestation onwards when exercise was carried out on the bicycle ergometer. These findings suggest that the bicycle ergometer is not a true non-weight-bearing exercise. Postural problems may have been implicated while cycling and leg oedema may have possibly increased weight of the lower limbs or interfered with mechanical efficiency. Heart rate and rated perceived exertion (RPE), as measured with the Borg scale, remained constant during gestation and reduced in the postpartum period.

South-Paul et al. (1988) reported a similar increase in physical fitness during pregnancy, although findings were statistically non-significant. They studied measurements of aerobic capacity ($VO_{2max}$) in healthy pregnant women at 20 and 30 weeks' gestation using a bicycle ergometer. Women, randomly assigned to either a non-exercising group ($n = 10$) or an exercise group ($n = 7$), trained for 1 hour four times per week under supervision. The exercise group demonstrated greater improvement in aerobic capacity than did the control group.

Clapp and Capeless (1991) investigated whether women ($n = 40$) could elicit a training effect during pregnancy. Healthy well-conditioned women ($n = 20$) participating in recreational exercise were studied for aerobic capacity before conception. Non-pregnant women ($n = 20$) acted as controls. After conception, women continued with their moderate–high exercise regime and were tested again during and after pregnancy. Non-pregnant participants remained unchanged in aerobic capacity whereas pregnant participants significantly increased their aerobic capacity during pregnancy. After delivery, aerobic capacity remained elevated between 12 and 20 weeks and was maintained at 38 weeks postpartum. Researchers concluded that a significant training effect may be possible when healthy recreational exercisers maintained a moderate–high exercise regime during pregnancy.

Kramer (2000) carried out a systematic review of research studies in this area. He concluded that regular aerobic exercise during pregnancy appeared to improve or maintain physical fitness. These findings suggest that pregnant women may be as trainable as their non-pregnant counterparts.

The most serious argument against the intensity of activity during pregnancy remains the concern in relation to the increase in body temperature, which is a normal response to physical activity (Leuzzi and Scoles 1996). Maternal hyperthermia and redistribution of blood to the working muscles and skin for thermoregulation may have an adverse effect on the development of the fetus (Huch and Erkkola 1990).

There is currently limited knowledge about fetal adaptability to thermal stress and to increased maternal heat production during exercise. It is postulated that changes in efficiency of heat dissipation, related to alterations in regional blood flow during pregnancy, enhances maternal cooling ability (Clapp et al. 1987). The woman's capacity for heat elimination during pregnancy may also be improved as a result of the increased vasodilatation response in the skin (Clapp 1991a, b; de Swiet 1991a). One possible explanation offered is that the relatively lower work intensity of work performance achieved by pregnant women is not sufficient to induce significant increases in body temperature.

In summary, numerous studies have investigated maternal adaptations to exercise during pregnancy. Studies suggest that exercise undertaken during pregnancy may improve or maintain physical fitness. The pregnant woman appears to be relatively well protected against hyperthermia in moderate exercise. Hyperthermia experienced by women during pregnancy is a particular area of concern because this may have an adverse effect on fetal development and growth. Further research is needed in this area to investigate maternal physiological effects during high intensity levels of exercise and prolonged episodes of moderate exercise.

## Fetal considerations

The fetus requires a continuous and adequate supply of oxygen and nutrients for its metabolism and growth. Severe, acute interference with fetal supply is likely to cause hypoxic damage, whereas milder more chronic reductions may result in suboptimal growth. Fetal heart rate (FHR) and oxygen consumption are physiological variables that may represent only temporary adjustments. Therefore, these factors provide limited information about whether fetal tolerance is exceeded and when irreversible damage may have occurred.

A reduction in the uterine blood flow during exercise could imply that the blood supply to the fetus will also be compromised (Riemann and Kanstrup Hansen 2000). This remains a controversial issue when comparing animal and human studies. Several lines of evidence, based on animal studies, suggest that the fetus may experience transient hypoxia during maternal aerobic exercise as a result of redistribution of blood from the viscera to the working muscles.

In early animal studies, Clapp (1980) reported no appreciable changes in uterine blood flow in pregnant ewes not exercised to exhaustion on a treadmill, in contrast to a decrease (28%) in uterine blood flow in pregnant ewes exercised to exhaustion. The fetuses showed signs of compromise as a result of reduced uterine blood flow, although this reduction was well tolerated. The investigations of Lotgering et al. (1983) found that uterine blood flow in sheep was reduced by up to 25% when exercise was both prolonged and strenuous. Findings suggest that the reduction in uterine blood flow in sheep was adequately compensated for by various mechanisms to maintain uterine oxygen uptake (Lotgering et al. 1983, 1984, 1985).

Measurement of heart rate provides a valuable tool in assessing fetal well-being. Typical changes in FHR are known to reflect hypoxic and non-hypoxic stress, hypoxia or asphyxia, and sympathetic and parasympathetic activity. The human FHR response to maternal exercise has been studied repeatedly since Hon and Wohlgemuth (1961) introduced it as a clinical test for 'uteroplacental insufficiency'. Monitoring of FHR is a non-invasive ultrasonographic technique used in clinical obstetrics to detect 'fetal distress' and to predict outcome of the fetus. Severe bradycardia (FHR < 100 beats/min), tachycardia (FHR > 160 beats/min), loss of variability (bandwidth < 5 beats/min) and the presence of 'late' decelerations (occurring outwith a contraction) are empirically associated with fetal distress and poor fetal outcome. Positive indications of fetal well-being and outcome are suggested by good variability and accelerations in FHR (Sweet and Tiran 1997).

A number of studies reported the findings on measurements of FHR response and fetal breathing movements in pregnant women before, during and after exercise. All findings suggest that, although there was some kind of fetal response to exercise, it remains unclear whether the fetus experiences hypoxic stress (Riemann and Kanstrup Hansen 2000). It is often technically difficult to assess blood flow and changes during exercise, so the interpretation of results made after exercise should be treated with caution. It is possible that uterine blood flow might very rapidly return to, or above, the pre-exercise level.

An increase in FHR is a normal response to maternal exercise. A number of early and more recent studies demonstrate that the FHR response to maternal aerobic exercise involves a gradual increase in FHR up to 20 beats/min during exercise and returns to pre-exercise baselines within 20 min after the exercise (Dressendorfer and Goodlin 1980; Hauth et al. 1982; Collings and Curet 1985; Carpenter et al. 1988; Wolfe et al. 1989b; Clapp et al. 1993; Webb et al. 1994).

Under most conditions, the human FHR directly reflects fetal cardiac output. The Frank–Starling mechanism, which regulates cardiac output, is not well developed in the fetus. However, some early and recent studies of FHR response support the hypothesis that some fetuses may experience hypoxia during or after maternal aerobic exercise. Fetal bradycardia has the potential to affect the fetus adversely if it was sustained during exercise or if there was a delay after exercise in the recovery of FHR to pre-exercise levels.

Results of other investigations suggest the presence of episodes of fetal bradycardia during and after maternal exercise (Dale et al. 1982; Jovanovic et al. 1988; Watson et al. 1991; Manders et al. 1997). Watson et al. (1991) noted six episodes of marked transient fetal brady-cardia in 15% of subjects after vigorous exercise. Bung et al. (1991), in a case study of a professional athlete, recorded fetal bradycardia during strenuous exercise, but did not record any changes to FHR during submaximal maternal exercise. Manders et al. (1997) conclude that moderate-to-heavy exercise clearly affects the human fetus with signs of transient fetal impairment after heavy exercise.

In summary, evidence based on animal and human studies suggests that the fetus may experience transient hypoxia during maternal exercise. There is concern that this may have adverse effects on the fetus. Numerous studies have documented fetal physiological response, especially in FHR response to maternal exercise. Findings suggest that FHR changes during maternal exercise are transient and do not inter-fere with normal fetal development and growth. As a reduction in FHR is assumed to reflect fetal distress, it is advisable that further more detailed study is carried out in this field.

## Clinical outcome

There has been growing concern that physical activity undertaken during pregnancy may result in pre-term labour (Reimann and Kanstrup Hansen 2000). Pre-term delivery occurs before 37 completed weeks of the 40-week gestation period and may compromise the well-being of the newborn (Sweet and Tiran 1997). High levels of circu-lating noradrenaline were recorded during exercise (Gorski 1985) and theoretically these levels may stimulate uterine contractions and result in pre-term labour (Zuspan et al. 1962).

A number of early and more recent studies conclude that physical activity during pregnancy does not influence the incidence of pre-term labour (Pomerance et al. 1974; Veille et al. 1985; Clapp 1989, 1990; Beckmann and Beckmann 1990; Botkin and Driscoll 1991).

Veille et al. (1985) reported that exercise did not increase post-exercise uterine activity during the last 8 weeks of pregnancy. Clapp (1989) compared early pregnancy outcomes of physically fit, active, pregnant women who continued aerobic exercise ($n = 90$) with a control group ($n = 29$) who were intermittently active. He concludes that exercise, maintained at a high intensity level during the period of conception and early pregnancy, does not appear to alter early pregnancy outcomes. Evidence from a similar study concludes that exercise does not trigger pre-term labour in healthy women ($n = 87$) who regularly exercised during pregnancy (Clapp 1990).

A previous retrospective study reported that exercise during pregnancy was not associated with pre-term delivery among Olympic athletes (Zaharieva 1972) and more recently a case study of an élite athlete during pregnancy supported these findings (Bung et al. 1991). In contrast, Clapp and Dickstein (1984) carried out a prospective study of pregnant women who participated in exercise or were sedentary. They reported that women ($n = 29$) who continued to exercise after 28 weeks had a significantly shorter gestation than either those women ($n = 47$) who had ceased exercise before 28 weeks' gestation or sedentary women ($n = 149$).

Mayberry et al. (1992) evaluated the short-term effects of exercise on uterine activity in women ($n = 10$) who were classified as being at 'high risk' of pre-term labour. Results indicated that there were minimal changes in the frequency of uterine contractions after a protocol of conditioning exercises. They recommended that future research was needed to evaluate short- and long-term effects of exercise on high-risk pregnancies.

A number of epidemiological studies have associated risk with various kinds of occupations and activities, whereas others regard prolonged standing as the possible critical factor for risk of pre-term labour.

Misra et al. (1998) conducted a study on a cohort of low-income women to determine the effect of physical activity on the risk of pre-term birth. Current recommendations regarding leisure time and daily living activities were supported by the findings. However, the two activities of climbing stairs and walking appeared to increase the risk of pre-term delivery among low-income women. Similar findings were reported by Homer et al. (1990), Klebanoff et al. (1990), Grisso et al. (1992) and Hedegaard et al. (1995).

Findings from a prospective cohort of women ($n = 4259$) suggest that standing and walking at work during the second trimester of pregnancy may present a particular risk for pre-term delivery (Hedegaard et al. 1995). In a small study, physical activities such as prolonged standing, heavy lifting or structured exercise did not appear to affect uterine contraction rates in a cohort ($n = 81$) of low-risk pregnant women using continuous ambulatory cardiotocography for 72 hours on three occasions during pregnancy. However, walking and climbing stairs did show a significant and persistent effect on uterine activity during the third trimester of pregnancy (Grisso et al. 1992).

Klebanoff et al. (1990) studied a cohort of pregnant women ($n$ = 7101) prospectively to evaluate employment- and non-employment-related physical activity. They reported an association between prolonged periods of standing with a modestly increased risk of pre-term delivery. No association was found among heavy work, exercise and pre-term delivery. However, Homer et al. (1990) conclude that women who undertook jobs characterized by high levels of physical exertion experienced a higher rate of pre-term labour and low birth-weight (< 2.5 kg) babies. Work-related high physical exertion may be deleterious to pregnancy because the blood supply to the uterus may possibly be halved and increased 20-fold to leg muscles (Chamberlain 1991).

In general, the available data suggest that there are no important effects of exercise on shortening of gestation, which should be reassuring to healthy women who wish to exercise during pregnancy.

There is a belief that exercise during pregnancy promotes physical fitness, which may ease labour and delivery. In this respect, many women hope that regular physical activity during pregnancy will prepare them to cope more efficiently with the exhausting early days of motherhood. It would be logical to expect labour to be facilitated by improved physical conditioning and improved function of specific muscles employed in the active stage of labour. However, labour is a very complex process and many factors such as parity, maternal age, fetal size and position, and the use of analgesic medications could alter its course (Sweet and Tiran 1997).

Recent research has focused on clinical issues related to the outcome of labour and delivery. Existing studies have used the duration of the stages of labour as an indication of the difficulty of labour and the The Apgar score for assessment of the newborn. Labour involves three stages: the first stage is passive and begins from the onset of regular, rhythmic, uterine contractions until full dilatation of the cervix; the second stage is defined from full dilatation of the cervix until delivery of the baby; and the third stage occurs from delivery of the baby until expulsion of the placenta and membranes (Sweet and Tiran 1997). The Apgar score is a traditional way of assessing the general condition of the newborn. It is a numerical score devised by Dr Virginia Apgar (1953) and grades five clinical features of the infant at 1, 5 and 10 min after birth (cited in Robertson 1993). Higher scores indicate a positive outcome for the newborn to adapt to extrauterine life, whereas lower scores indicate poorer outcome with potential problems of varying degrees.

Research findings are varied in relation to the experiences of labour and delivery. Some researchers found no difference between women who exercised and control group women in the length of labour, type of delivery or the incidence of complications or fetal distress (Kupla et al. 1987; Lee 1996; Kardel and Kase 1998). In the study carried out by Kupla et al. (1987), primigravid women who exercised were found to have a significantly shorter active first stage of labour than non-exercising counterparts, although no difference was found between multigravid women. Other researchers reported that women who exercised experienced significantly shorter labours, a reduction in the incidence of obstetric complications (Clapp 1990; Botkin and Driscoll 1991; Wang and Apgar 1998), and a significant reduction in the incidence of surgical deliveries and length of stay in hospital (Hall and Kaufmann 1987).

There were noticeable differences in the research design and methods used in these studies. Botkin and Driscoll (1991) grouped women into non-exercising and exercising groups according to their exercise history in a retrospective study with women ($n = 44$) who had given birth in the preceding 7 months. Lee (1996) conducted a randomized controlled study of women ($n = 370$) who were assigned to a regular structured exercise programme or a control group, whereas Kardel and Kase (1998) investigated the effects of exercise with women ($n = 42$) who self-selected into medium- and high-intensity exercise programmes throughout and after pregnancy.

In a large study, Hall and Kaufmann (1987) studied birth outcome from clinical records in a large group of pregnant women ($n = 845$) undertaking aerobic conditioning. Participants were divided into four groups consisting of one control group ($n = 393$) who did not exercise and three exercise groups participating in low ($n = 82$), medium ($n = 309$) and high levels ($n = 61$) of exercise. An interesting prospective study of healthy well-conditioned athletes carried out by Clapp (1990) included recreational runners ($n = 67$) and aerobic dancers ($n = 64$). The exercise group ($n = 87$) continued to exercise throughout pregnancy at a high level of performance and women ($n = 44$) who spontaneously stopped exercise in the first trimester of pregnancy were allocated to the control group.

Many of the researchers recognized limitations within the studies, in relation to the research design, sample size, self-selection of participants not being representative of the general population of pregnant women, and duration and timing of the study.

Physical activity increases the secretion of endogenous opiates and abnormally high amounts of β-endorphins have been measured in the blood plasma of exercising participants. β-endorphins are known to have an opiate effect on the central nervous system (CNS), and this has resulted in much speculation in recent years about their role in pain perception. There is agreement in the literature regarding the increased secretion of β-endorphins during labour (Raisanen et al. 1984). It is reasonable to hypothesize that, if labour is considered to be a combination of intense physical exercise and bouts of acute painful stimulation, the stimulus for endogenous opiate secretion will be maximal during this period. Varassi et al. (1989) compared multigravid women in a control group with multigravid women who exercised during pregnancy. They concluded that exercise conditioning during pregnancy appeared to be beneficial in reducing both perception of pain and stress levels during labour.

Research findings in relation to birthweight and Apgar scores of babies at birth are inconsistent. Many early and more recent researchers agree that there is no difference between women who exercise during pregnancy and sedentary women in relation to birthweight and Apgar scores (Collings et al. 1983; Slavin 1988; Botkin and Driscoll 1991; Rose et al. 1991; Sternfield et al. 1995; Lee 1996; Kardel and Kase 1998). In contrast, Hall and Kaufmann (1987) reported that babies born to mothers in the high exercise group had higher Apgar scores than babies born to mothers in the other groups.

Some investigators have found that women who were moderately trained had significantly heavier babies than highly trained or nontrained women (Hatch et al. 1993; Bell et al. 1995). Other researchers have reported that babies born to exercising women were significantly lighter than babies born to non-exercising women from control groups (Clapp and Dickstein 1984; Clapp and Capeless 1990; Bell et al. 1995; Clapp et al. 1998a).

Clapp et al. (1998a) investigated the babies of women who had continued to exercise during pregnancy (n = 52) compared with infants (n = 52) of women from a control group. At birth, the infants of exercising women weighed less and had less body fat. However, at 1 year of age all morphometric parameters were similar, and normal growth and development occurred during the first year of life.

Bell et al. (1995) assessed the effect on birthweight of a continuing programme of vigorous exercise into late pregnancy. 'Potential exercisers' (n = 58) continued to exercise during pregnancy and were compared with a control group of women (n = 48) who did not exercise on a regular basis. Women in the exercise group who participated in more than four sessions of vigorous exercise per week at 25 weeks' gestation were reported to have babies with a mean birthweight of 315 g lower than those in the control group. Women who were moderately trained had babies with significantly higher birthweight.

Clapp and Capeless (1990) prospectively monitored maternal body composition during pregnancy (n = 132) and infant body composition and birthweight. It was noted that women who exercised ($n = 77$) during pregnancy gave birth to infants 500 g lighter in weight than infants born to women in the control group ($n = 55$) who did not plan to exercise. The difference in birthweight was primarily the result of a reduction in fetal fat mass in women who continued to exercise through late gestation. This did not create clinical difficulty in the neonatal period and it was speculated that, if the leanness continued, there could be a potential long-term cardiovascular benefit in later life. There is a potential problem that the difference in birthweight could put the pre-term infant at greater risk of morbidity and mortality.

Pivarnik (1998) concludes, from a review of the literature, that there was a mixed relationship between the potential effects of maternal physical activity and birthweight. Current evidence suggests that participation in moderate-to-vigorous activity throughout pregnancy may enhance birthweight whereas more severe regimes may result in lighter infants. The reason for this could be attributed to an increase in placental size as a result of the training that leads to an improved blood flow to the fetus (Clapp and Rizk 1992; Jackson et al. 1995). Careful caloric calculations and quantification in chronic exercise are needed before further conclusions can be drawn.

Lokey et al. (1991) carried out a meta-analytical study examining the effects of physical exercise on pregnancy outcomes. The studies reviewed involved 2314 pregnant women, 1357 experimental and 957 control participants. Overall results indicate that there were no apparent adverse effects of exercise in the studies reviewed. They suggest that limitations should not be imposed on the level of exercise undertaken during pregnancy.

Findings conclude that healthy, pregnant and well-conditioned women may take part in exercise during pregnancy without compromising fetal growth and development, as judged by birthweight or complications during the course of pregnancy and labour. However, findings in the area of labour and birth outcome remain controversial and further research is required to allow conclusions to be established.

In summary, recent research has focused on the effects of exercise on pregnancy and birth outcomes. The literature suggests that exercise during pregnancy does not influence the incidence of pre-term labour. Numerous studies have reported on the clinical issues surrounding the process of labour and delivery in relation to duration of labour, mode of delivery and the incidence of obstetric complications. Findings in relation to the effects of exercise on labour and delivery outcomes remain inconclusive. This is mainly the result of studies conducted with small sample size and self-selected participants, which makes it difficult to generalize the findings to other pregnant women. Other studies have focused on the effects that maternal exercise may have on birthweight and neonatal well-being. Findings agree that there are no adverse effects to neonatal well-being at birth. However, findings in relation to birthweight tend to be controversial. Further research needs to be conducted with large well-controlled studies to allow detailed investigation of the effects of exercise on pregnancy and birth outcome.

### Maternal muscle and skeletal considerations

Pregnant women need to be cautious when undertaking any physical activity during pregnancy because they experience increased laxity of their ligaments, resulting from increased production of the hormone relaxin (Dumas and Reid 1997). Change in joint laxity during pregnancy is analogous to that in someone who has just had surgery on the joints and ligaments (Artal Mittlemark et al. 1991a). These factors contribute to pregnant women being more prone than normal to soft tissue and skeletal injury (Huch and Erkkola 1990). During pregnancy, the relaxation of ligaments, combined with lordosis, changes in the centre of gravity and weight gain, should increase stress in most joints. Weight-bearing exercises and sudden movements generate significant torque and sheer stress to the joints. Despite this apparent increased susceptibility, there are no reports of any increase in injury rate when exercise is performed during pregnancy (Clapp 1994, 2000).

The encumbrance and additional weight of the fetus could constitute additional stress in any physical activity involving weight support. Spinal and pelvic insufficiency is common during pregnancy. As a result of these factors, there is growing concern about the incidence of low back pain experienced by women during and after pregnancy.

Berg et al. (1988) carried out a large prospective study of pregnant women (n = 862) in Sweden. Low back pain was reported for short periods of time during pregnancy by 49% of women and back pain was experienced for longer than 6 months of pregnancy in 6% of all women. Reports of severe pain in 9% of women, classified as medically unfit for work, resulted in referral to an orthopaedic surgeon for orthoneurological examination. The most common diagnosis was sacroiliac joint instability. Backache tended to remain a problem after delivery in 60% of these women who had experienced severe pain during pregnancy. However, backache was resolved in all women by 12 months postpartum.

Parsons (1994) recommends that, during early pregnancy, women should be encouraged to do some gentle exercise to offset some of the mechanical strain that arises with postural changes as pregnancy progresses. Hall and Kaufmann (1987) found that participants who had stopped exercising for longer than 2 weeks reported recurrence of common aches and pains, especially low back pain. Andrews and O'Neill (1994) suggest that pelvic (hip) tilt exercises appear to be effective in reducing ligament pain intensity and duration.

There is currently little specific information available about the incidence of sports injuries during pregnancy. Anecdotal reports suggest that there are few problems in highly trained, well-conditioned athletes who maintain their endurance activities into the second trimester (Jarrett and Spellacy 1983; Cohen et al. 1989).

Debate surrounds the factors contributing to subsequent weakness of the pelvic floor muscles after vaginal delivery. As a result of traumatic damage, many women experience some degree of urinary incontinence after childbirth, although between 60% and 80% of problems do regress spontaneously (Candy 1994). Some authors suggest that exercise is beneficial to assist the muscles in returning to their pre-pregnant condition and to minimize pelvic floor damage during delivery (Henderson 1983; Shephard 1983; Gordon and Logue 1985; Morkvid and Bo 1996). These exercises were originally designed to increase the elasticity and tonicity of the perineum and to prevent perineal tears during delivery of the baby. No scientific evidence is available to support this theory, and research in the mid-1980s questions the effectiveness of this type of exercise. Sleep and Grant (1987) suggest that pelvic floor exercises are of limited value in preventing damage, although others suggest that weakness after vaginal delivery results from damage to the innervation of pelvic floor muscles rather than stretching of the muscles (Snooks et al. 1984).

Gordon and Logue (1985) recommend that regular general exercise improves the tone of the pelvic floor muscles. Valancogne and Galaup (1993) suggest that perineal exercise, abdominal exercise and physical activity are not contradictory, but complementary, and should be adapted to the individual woman.

## Psychological benefits of exercise during pregnancy

Psychological benefits of exercise during pregnancy are important to women to help them cope with the changes brought about by pregnancy. These include anatomical and physiological changes, physical discomforts, lifestyle changes and other social factors (Raphael-Leff 1991; Clement 1998).

Many reports have investigated the proposed 'mental health' benefits of exercise with normal and clinical populations. Research studies have investigated the emotional and cognitive consequences resulting from involvement in an exercise programme. Findings indicate that physical activity is positively associated with lower levels of depression, anxiety, more positive moods and increased self-esteem, and feelings of well-being (Stephens 1988; Moses et al. 1989; Steptoe et al. 1989; Crammer et al. 1991). However, there are only a few reported studies investigating the psychological effects of exercise during pregnancy.

Wallace et al. (1986) compared subjective responses to exercise in women participating in aerobic exercise during pregnancy ($n = 37$) with a group of non-exercising women ($n = 22$). Women in the exercise group had participated in exercise for at least 4 weeks before data collection at 27 weeks of pregnancy. The groups did not differ significantly with respect to age, gestational age, parity or weight gain during pregnancy. A physical discomfort checklist was specifically designed to measure the individual's perception of the frequency and intensity of minor symptoms occurring during pregnancy. Exercising participants had scores, which indicated higher self-esteem than the control group. The exercising group had a significantly lower incidence of overall physical symptoms and of backache, shortness of breath, fatigue, headache and hot flushes. A significant inverse relationship was also observed between the overall incidence of physical symptoms and the total duration of exercise performed during the third trimester of pregnancy. The researchers recognized that self-selection of the participants may have influenced the results.

Similar findings were reported by Hall and Kaufmann (1987) who carried out a large retrospective study to evaluate the effects of a combined programme of aerobic and strength-conditioning exercises on self-image, reductions in physical complaints and relief of tension in women after childbirth. Participants were divided into either a control group ($n = 393$), or high ($n = 82$), medium ($n = 309$) and low ($n = 61$) intensity exercise groups based on attendance at supervised classes. Comfort was assessed from subjective reports by the participants and included tension level, general physical discomfort and sense of well-being. All exercise participants reported improved self-image, reduced tension and a decrease in physical discomforts during the time of participation. Multigravid women reported a more rapid postpartum recovery than previous pregnancies. Horns et al. (1996) conclude, from their study, that those women who engaged in active exercise during the third trimester of pregnancy experienced fewer of the common disorders of pregnancy. Heffernan (2000) suggests that exercise may actually decrease the associated discomforts of pregnancy and increase maternal fitness and well-being.

Slavin et al. (1988) conducted a retrospective ($n = 195$) and prospective study ($n = 182$) to investigate subjective responses to exercise during pregnancy. From their findings, they conclude that women perceived that regular exercise during pregnancy enabled them to have control over their bodies at a time of profound bodily changes. The authors suggest that exercise continued during pregnancy is an aid to maintaining a positive self-image and providing women with an opportunity for relaxation.

More recently, Koniak-Griffin (1994) studied the effects of participation in an aerobic exercise programme over a 6-week period for adolescent pregnant females between 14 and 20 years of age. Participants in the exercise group were observed to have a decrease in depressive symptoms over time and an increase in total self-esteem. Significant differences were found between the exercise group when compared with a comparison group who also reported an increase in physical discomforts associated with pregnancy. The researchers suggest that exercise during pregnancy promotes psychological wellbeing.

Koltyn and Schultes (1997) studied a self-selected group of women (n = 20) who had delivered a baby within the past year. Mood changes in the postpartum period were studied after exercise and quiet rest periods. Results indicated that 'state anxiety' and depression decreased significantly after exercise and quiet rest. Exercise was associated with significant decreases in total mood disturbances as well as significant increases in vigour in the exercising women.

In summary, there is general agreement within the literature that exercise during pregnancy has a beneficial effect on psychological wellbeing of women. Benefits reported include improved feelings of 'wellbeing', reduced anxiety and tension, improved mood, increased self-image and coping abilities. Literature in this area is limited and further research is needed to confirm these current findings.

## Gaps in the literature

There are many legal and ethical aspects to be considered when investigating humans in relation to exercise during pregnancy. Therefore, a great deal of research has been undertaken with humans in supervised laboratory conditions or with animal models. Experimental paradigms and species difference in the physiological response make it difficult to apply any findings to the human condition (Mottola 1996).

The two major deficits in published studies are the lack of prospective, adequately controlled, experimental design and inadequate quantification of physical activity. Limitations with the methodologies of many of the studies discussed include small sample sizes, self-selected groups, sparse or intermittent episodes of exercise, poor adherence to the exercise programmes, limited monitoring of variables and retrospective data collection over varying periods of time.

In many trials, the method of treatment allocation either is not described or has involved non-random selection. Most did not specify the number of participants, compliance with the exercise programme, the reasons for loss of participants or any follow-up studies. Many studies had eliminated those women who developed complications and therefore did not report data on either the number of affected participants or the resulting conditions or outcomes.

Some of the studies attempted to generalize findings from exercise programmes of different levels of intensities for different periods of time and to relate these findings to the effects of exercise on pregnancy outcome. The assumption that exercise conducted at different intensities for different periods of time all have the same effect on pregnancy and birth outcome is a major concern.

There was the suspicion that some researchers may have an element of bias towards the positive outcome of pregnancy by women undertaking exercise. Many of the studies discussed have indicated that women who exercised during pregnancy can have a positive outcome to their pregnancy. However, the validity of any overall conclusion about the effects on pregnancy remains questionable.

Design of controlled investigations on psychological effects of physical conditioning during pregnancy is troublesome because adherence to exercise is difficult to maintain during long-term prospective studies. Psychological variables are easily affected by participants' attitudes and beliefs, and studies discussed allowed group selection that may have improved adherence to the assigned exercise group, although results may be invalidated as a result of selection bias.

Healthy pregnant women who engage in regular aerobic exercise in pregnancy are likely to be more fit than their more sedentary peers, but knowledge of the risks and benefits for themselves and their infants will require studies that are better controlled than the many trials discussed within the review.

There is a wealth of research evidence available in relation to the physiological effects of exercise during pregnancy, but to date there is very little research that considers the psychological aspects during the process of childbirth. The benefits of exercise on psychological wellbeing of non-pregnant women are well documented in the literature, but there are few studies documenting the psychological effects of exercise during and after pregnancy.

It is evident from reviewing the literature that well-controlled human studies are needed to provide information on the effects of exercise on pregnancy and pregnancy outcome, and the impact on the physiological and psychological well-being of the woman. Unfortunately, the available data are insufficient to show important risks or benefits for mother and baby, although theoretical advantages of exercise during pregnancy are positive and worthy of further investigation. In view of the current trend towards a more physically active society, health professionals have an obligation to investigate, design and promote activities that are safe and maintain maternal and fetal well-being.

## Summary of the literature review

Women now regard exercise as part of their normal life and many wish to continue to exercise during pregnancy. The physical and psychological benefits of exercise are well documented, and for many years it has been suggested that women could enjoy these benefits during pregnancy. This suggestion has raised many concerns that the impact of exercise on pregnancy may have an adverse effect on the normal progress of pregnancy and the developing fetus. A wealth of scientific research has now been undertaken to investigate the physiological effects of exercise on maternal and fetal well-being and pregnancy and birth outcomes. More studies investigating psychological well-being are emerging in the literature.

Over the past 30 years, a significant body of evidence supports the hypothesis that healthy women can perform acute exercise of moderate intensity and duration without jeopardizing fetal well-being. Findings agree that maternal exercise is well tolerated by the fetus. There are no published reports of fetal compromise or adverse outcome of pregnancy as a result of maternal exercise.

It is agreed that women who exercise during pregnancy do experience both physiological and psychological benefits. Women experience improved stamina, physical fitness, muscle tone, and improved feelings of physical and mental well-being. Findings from the literature suggest that exercise does not have any influence on the incidence of pre-term labour or any adverse effects to the fetus. In fact, there is evidence to suggest that the fetus can tolerate physiological effects of maternal exercise. Findings remain inconclusive in relation to the effects of exercise on pregnancy and birth outcomes. It is, generally, considered to be safe for healthy women to undertake regular moderate exercise during pregnancy without any risk to pregnancy or the baby.

Research studies involving human pregnancy studies have many legal and ethical considerations. As a result, animal studies have been used to investigate the physiological effects of pregnancy and there is difficulty in trying to generalise these findings to pregnant women. Studies undertaken with humans tend to have flaws in the research design such as self-selected participants and small sample size. Well-controlled studies are required to investigate in detail the effects of exercise during pregnancy. The potential impact of occasional, regular and prolonged exercise during pregnancy on outcomes of clinical importance for the mother and infants remains unknown.

# The present study

The study used a two-group randomized controlled trial to investigate and compare the effect of a structured exercise programme on healthy women during and after their first pregnancy. The control group of participants continued with the existing antenatal education programme offered to prepare women for pregnancy, labour and the transition to parenthood. In addition, the women in the intervention group participated in a structured exercise programme during and after pregnancy. Participants were studied from 12 weeks of pregnancy until 4 months after delivery of the baby.

The outcome measures focused mainly on psychological indicators of well-being. These included how the women felt about themselves and their bodies, how well they felt they could cope, and attitudes to marital relationships, sex, pregnancy and the baby. Pregnancy and birth outcomes were also investigated, in addition to the amount of physical activity undertaken throughout the study.

The research design and methodology of the present study addressed some of the gaps identified in the review of scientific studies:

- The study is a randomized controlled trial
- Participants were healthy primigravid women with uncomplicated pregnancies
- Although small, the sample size was sufficient to gain significance with statistical tests
- The study followed participants from early pregnancy until 20 weeks postpartum
- Measurement tools are validated and reliable
- Statistical testing was rigorous and undertaken at identified times during the study
- Indicators of psychological well-being were investigated
- The structured exercise programme remained consistent throughout the study in both format and instructor
- Frequency and type of physical activity were recorded for all participants
- Information available from participants who dropped out of the study was investigated.

**Statement of aims**

The study aimed to compare an intervention and control group of healthy women during and after their first pregnancy. Comparisons were made in early pregnancy (12–16 weeks), late pregnancy (36–40 weeks) and after pregnancy (12–16 weeks) in relation to the following:

- Psychological 'well-being' in terms of perceptions of coping assets (positive psychological well-being), perceptions of coping deficits (negative psychological well-being) and postnatal emotional well-being and depression
- Perceptions of physical well-being
- Perceptions of somatic symptoms experienced
- Perceptions of body image
- Maternal attitudes to marital relationships and sex
- Maternal attitudes to pregnancy and baby
- Pregnancy outcomes in terms of: length of gestation, duration of labour and type of delivery
- Birth outcomes in terms of: Apgar score, birthweight and neonatal complications
- Maternal medical or obstetric conditions experienced
- Physical activity levels in early pregnancy
- Physical activity participation
- Drop-out rate from the study.

This chapter has provided a review of the literature covering many aspects related to exercise and pregnancy. It has included an overview of exercise and the associated physical, psychological and health benefits to the healthy individual, and the physiological and psychological changes of pregnancy. An overview of the history of exercise in obstetrics is presented and, finally, a detailed review of scientific studies of exercise and pregnancy over the previous 30 years. A summary of the gaps in the literature is provided.

The purpose of providing this wide range of literature has been to enable the reader to develop more understanding of the complexity of the issues surrounding exercise and pregnancy. The aims of the present study have been outlined and the next chapter provides detail of how the research study was carried out.

# Chapter 3
# Research methodology

This chapter reports on the methodology of this study, in which the effects of a structured exercise programme were investigated with healthy women during and after their first pregnancy. The chapter is divided into three related sections, with each subsequent section providing the reader with additional and more explicit information about different aspects of the research methodology.

The first section provides a detailed account of the research design and methods used within the study. The overall aim is to provide a rationale for the methods used in explicit detail to allow the study to be replicated.

The second section describes the pilot study undertaken before the main study. This proved to be important and worthwhile because it allowed the initial methodology to be tested and evaluated. I would like to emphasize to the reader the important contribution made by the pilot study to the final research design. It was only on hindsight that this value was truly appreciated as I was eager to proceed with the main study. Time taken during this phase resulted in the final research design being more efficient and effective. This section should be of interest and value to those readers who are inexperienced in research.

The third section provides further more detailed information about the exercise programme designed for pregnancy and after birth. This includes the principles of the programme related to the anatomical and physiological changes experienced during pregnancy and after birth, the aim of the exercise components, precautions and recommendations, and guidelines for exercise. This section should be of interest to readers who want further information about the design of exercise programmes for pregnancy and after birth.

# Research design and methods

## Research design

The study was a randomized controlled trial of two groups of healthy women during and after their first pregnancy. The control group of participants continued with the existing antenatal care programme offered in Ayrshire to prepare women for pregnancy, childbirth, postpartum period and the transition to parenthood. In addition, participants allocated to the intervention group took part in a structured antenatal and postnatal exercise programme during and after pregnancy.

## Planning

Initially, a small multidisciplinary group of health professionals assisted in planning the study. This group included a physiotherapist, a midwife, an obstetric registrar, a midwifery sister from the antenatal clinic, an administrator, a consultant obstetrician and myself, the researcher. Individual members had knowledge and expertise in their own field of interest to assist in the development of the study. Once the planning stage was completed, both the midwifery sister and the consultant obstetrician remained in close liaison with the researcher throughout the study.

At this stage, careful consideration was given to the potential areas of concern identified by Steptoe (1992) when attempting to link physical activity and psychological well-being. These issues included: the appropriate measures of psychological experience; the factors that potentially confound studies of this topic; and the problem of the drop-out of participants from activity programmes.

The planning stage also consisted of locating a suitable venue for the exercise class, submitting applications for funding to support the cost of the study, and preparing the researcher to become qualified and experienced as an antenatal and postnatal exercise instructor.

Initially a pilot study was undertaken to evaluate and assess all aspects of the proposed methodology before undertaking the main study. The pilot study was designed for completion within one year. This aimed to gain an overview of the proposed methodology during each stage of the study. The pilot study is presented in more detail towards the end of this section.

## Main study participants

Participants were first-time prospective mothers who attended the antenatal clinic for the first antenatal appointment in early pregnancy, i.e. before 12 weeks' gestation.

Consultant obstetricians agreed the criteria for inclusion of participants into the study. Women who wished to participate in the study required the agreement of the consultant obstetrician responsible for their antenatal care. An ultrasound scan routinely performed during this appointment confirmed pregnancy and provided other obstetric assessment, which included the gestational age of the fetus.

Typical criteria for determining 'low-risk' pregnancy included:

- Healthy women having their first pregnancy, i.e. primigravid
- Singleton pregnancy
- Satisfactory medical history and ultrasound scan
- Satisfactory history of current pregnancy to date
- No reported history of
  - low lying placenta
  - previous obstetric history
  - threatened abortion
  - pre-existing chronic conditions, e.g. heart disease, respiratory conditions, epilepsy, diabetes mellitus, liver disease, and high blood pressure; these conditions are reported to be clear reasons to discourage the already 'at-risk' individual from exercising while pregnant (Carbon 1994).

Women did not continue with the exercise programme if they developed any complication or disorder during pregnancy that resulted in their transfer from midwifery to medical care, including:

- Threatened abortion
- Antepartum haemorrhage
- Intrauterine growth retardation
- Premature rupture of membranes
- High blood pressure/pre-eclampsia.

## Ethical permission

Ethical permission was sought and granted from the ethics committee of Ayrshire and Arran Health Board who have responsibility for monitoring research in the local maternity area. Emphasis from the committee was placed on the following ethical issues: the inclusion of obtaining informed consent from women to join the study; the obstetricians' agreement on the suitability of women for inclusion in the study; keeping participants well informed on all aspects of their allocated group (Sieber 1992); and ensuring adherence to the guidelines for the exercise programme.

Confidentiality of the participants in the study was maintained at all times (United Kingdom Central Council for Nursing, Midwifery, Health Visiting 1996) with strict compliance with the Data Protection Act in relation to personal and health details (Department of Health 1994, 1998). Permission was granted from North Ayrshire and Arran NHS Trust to review obstetric notes and the birth register to obtain relevant obstetric and medical information. Close liaison with obstetric staff was maintained when appropriate. Annual progress reports were forwarded to the ethics committee throughout the course of the study.

# Procedure

The data-gathering stage of the study was undertaken from August 1996 until December 1998. The main study was developed from the initial pilot study conducted. The duration of the study for each woman was approximately 52 weeks, i.e. from 8 weeks' gestation of pregnancy until 20 weeks after delivery of the baby.

## Recruitment

The medical clerkess and midwifery staff in the antenatal clinic conducted recruitment. On arrival for the first antenatal appointment, all primigravid women with no previous obstetric/medical history were initially given a brief letter requesting them to participate in a research study (no further information was given at this point). Women were recruited as participants in the study once consent was obtained and the obstetrician agreed that the obstetric criteria for entry to the study were met.

Initial consent to participate in the study was obtained from women at the first antenatal clinic appointment in early pregnancy, which was at approximately 8 weeks' gestation (see Appendix 1). The consultant obstetrician consented to each woman's suitability for the study during the first consultation with the woman and this was retained within the obstetric notes (see Appendix 2). Information leaflets about the allocated groups were issued to participants at the time of recruitment (see Appendices 6 and 7) and participants signed a further consent form for their group allocation (see Appendices 4 and 5). The researcher retained all consent forms from participants. Information letters were available for issue to individual general practitioners and midwives at the woman's request (see Appendix 3). Contact numbers were readily available to all participants and health professionals involved with the study. Participants were informed that, if they wished, they could leave the study at any time.

Recruitment of participants commenced in August 1996 and continued until November 1997 to ensure that an adequate number completed the study.

## Sample size

Sample size was estimated with the assistance of the statistician using the outcome indicators of perceptions of body image and of coping assets (positive psychological well-being) to determine the overall sample size necessary, in order to gain statistical significance. The range of possible scores for perception of body image was between 12 and 48. The typical score for the intervention group and control group in early pregnancy (i.e. between 12 and 16 weeks' gestation) was estimated to be 30 with subsequent scores in late pregnancy (i.e. between 36 and 40 weeks' gestation) estimated to be a score of 25 (–5) for the intervention group and a score of 20 (–10) for the control group. Based on this assumption, the study required a minimum of 30 participants to complete the study in each group for a power of 0.90 (Machin and Campbell 1991). Based on these calculations, and taking the drop-out rate from the pilot study into consideration, it was recommended that at least 50 participants should be recruited to each group.

## Randomization

Women were first identified on the appointment system as being primigravid women attending their first antenatal appointment. Written consent for participation in the study was obtained from both the women and the consultant obstetrician. The participants were then issued with a sealed and coded envelope that contained information about the study and their allocated group. They were aware of their allocated group only once the information pack had been opened. None of the staff involved in the recruitment process had knowledge of the group allocation. An equal number of sealed and coded information packs had been previously prepared by the researcher before recruitment of participants. These were issued to the antenatal clinic staff for distribution to the women. Each woman had an equal chance of being allocated to either of the two groups. Personal details and assigned code numbers were forwarded to the researcher. It was only at this point that the researcher had the relevant information to identify the participants to the allocated group.

## Control group

This group of participants continued with the existing antenatal education programme for the preparation of women for pregnancy, childbirth and the transition to parenthood. During pregnancy, this included routine regular obstetric care undertaken by midwives, general practitioners and consultant obstetricians. Routine midwifery care involved individualized care that was planned in partnership with the women and midwives. Women were routinely invited to attend structured classes for the preparation for pregnancy, labour and the transition to parenthood in either the hospital or community areas, workshops specifically for preparation for breast-feeding, and postnatal reunion and support groups. Aquanatal classes were an optional extra and classes were offered by most of the local leisure centres in conjunction with maternity service providers.

The information pack for participants in the control group included the following:

- A consent form to participate in the study (see Appendix 4)
- An information leaflet giving details of the control group (see Appendix 6)
- A letter giving details of the information required (see Appendix 9)
- A questionnaire booklet for completion in early pregnancy (see Appendix 10)
- Activity diary sheets (see Appendix 11)
- Contact number for the researcher.

Participants were not given any information about the structured exercise programme, although they were free to continue with their usual leisure-time activities. They were given information about additional activities and were asked to complete an activity diary for any episodes of physical activity (see Appendix 11). This was intended to help participants summarize information about all episodes of physical activity undertaken, in terms of the type, duration and frequency of physical activity. It provided information about the episodes of activity that could be divided into appropriate classifications of exercise, i.e. brisk walking, cycling, strength training, yoga, and other structured exercise classes such as aerobics and aquanatal. A stamped addressed envelope was provided for the return of information for the early pregnancy data collection point, i.e. consent form, completed initial questionnaire booklet and activity diary. Participants were encouraged to contact the researcher to discuss other physical activities that they either wished to participate in or had undertaken for their possible inclusion in the study.

Participants and babies in the control group were invited to a 'postnatal reunion' on completion of the study. The aim of this reunion was to thank them for their contribution to the study and finalize collation of relevant data.

## Intervention group

This group continued with the existing antenatal education programme for the preparation of women for pregnancy, childbirth and the transition to parenthood, in addition to participating in a structured antenatal and postnatal exercise programme. The exercise programme was designed to consider the anatomical and physiological changes of pregnancy with adherence to current guidelines.

The information pack for participants in the intervention group included the following:

- A consent form to participate in the study (see Appendix 5)
- An information leaflet with details of the intervention group (see Appendix 7)
- A questionnaire booklet for completion in early pregnancy (see Appendix 10)
- A letter giving details of the information required
- Activity diary sheets (see Appendix 11)
- Details of the venue for the intervention group with a map for directions
- Contact number for the researcher.

Participants were given information about additional forms of activity and were asked to complete an activity diary for any episodes of physical activity (see Appendix 11). This was intended to help them to summarize the information about additional physical activity undertaken in terms of the type, duration and frequency of physical activity. It provided information about the episodes of activity that could be divided into appropriate classifications of exercise, i.e. brisk walking, cycling, strength training, yoga, and other structured exercise classes such as aerobics and aquanatal. A stamped addressed envelope was provided for return of information for the early pregnancy data collection point, i.e. consent form, completed initial questionnaire booklet and activity diary.

Participants were also asked to sign a register of attendance at the structured exercise classes (see Appendix 13). This was intended to provide an overall total of all structured exercise classes attended at the end of the study. Participants could also take the opportunity at the exercise class to record other physical activities undertaken, in addition to the structured antenatal and postnatal exercise class provided.

Again, women and babies in the intervention group were invited to a 'postnatal reunion' on completion of the study. The aim of this reunion was to thank them for their contribution to the study and finalize collation of relevant data.

**Exercise programme**

This was a specially designed programme that complied with the guidelines of the American College of Obstetricians and Gynecologists (ACOG) for exercise during pregnancy and the postpartum period (cited in Artal Mittlemark et al. 1991c). The exercise programme was based on the London Central YMCA (1992) programme for exercise during and after pregnancy which has been endorsed by the Royal College of Midwives and the Association of Chartered Physiotherapists Specialising in Obstetrics & Gynaecology. The design of the exercise programme followed sound ergonomic principles as demonstrated by Gaskill (1992). It considered the anatomical, physiological and structural changes of pregnancy, and the possible impact of exercise on these changes.

The researcher was the instructor at all the structured exercise classes during the study. The aim of the programme was to provide exercise at moderate intensity. The intensity of the exercise undertaken by participants during the aerobic component of the exercise programme was monitored to assess the adequacy and severity of their aerobic activity by two different methods, i.e. assessment of heart rate by participants recording their own pulse rate and 'ratings of perceived exertion' (RPE) based on Borg's category scale. The value of using the heart rate as a monitoring tool for exercise intensity has been questioned. The original ACOG guidelines of 140 beats/min have been adopted as the maximum heart rate for women exercising during pregnancy. During pregnancy submaximal heart rates can be variable and this results in target heart rates being unpredictable. For this study, heart rate was used as a guide only. Intensity was assessed by combining heart rate with RPE and the 'talk test'.

The preferred method of assessment was monitoring of heart rate by participants recording their radial or carotid pulse rates at times of peak aerobic activity. Heart rates were monitored to ensure that pregnant participants did not have heart rates higher than 140 beats/min. Participants were informed of the target heart rate. Individual information, instruction and practice were given to enable them to become familiar with locating and recording their pulse rates. Heart rates were recorded for 30 seconds during the aerobic component of the exercise programme. This heart rate was subsequently doubled to ensure that heart rate per minute was within the target range for each participant. Those who reported a heart rate above the target rate were asked to reduce their exercise level, and the heart rate was recorded again to recheck that the rate was within the target range. Participants working under their target rate were asked to increase their exercise level.

Participants were also given information and instruction on assessing the adequacy and severity of RPE based on Borg's category scale during the aerobic exercise programme. The RPE scale is reported to equate subjective feelings of effort with numerical values derived from a standardized scale (see Appendix 14). The RPE scale has been most commonly used to assess difficulty of physical tasks by asking individuals to estimate their effort during physical exertion (Dunbar 1991), and has been shown to be valid in terms of productivity (Glass et al. 1992). It is a simple method to follow once individuals are familiar with the use of the scale. However, it has been suggested that pregnant participants may consistently underestimate their rate of actual physical exertion when using RPE scales, even when they are familiar with this method of assessment (O'Neill et al. 1992). However, this 'simple to use' visual scale provided an alternative to recording heart rate only when it was identified to be a problem for individuals to locate and record pulse rate during aerobic exercise. Large posters of the RPE scale were readily visible at the exercise class and participants were also given a smaller card detailing the scale for individual use. They were asked to estimate their perceived exertion rate (RPE) according to the scale during aerobic activity. The rating of '6' represents the participant's exercise 'at rest' whereas '20' represents the hardest level of activity. The recommended 50–60% of maximal functional capacity correlates with 13–14 on the RPE scale. In addition, an assistant at the classes recorded pulse rates to ensure that heart rate was within the target range. However, participants were encouraged to continue to practise recording their heart rate in order to transfer to this method when they felt confident to do so. Both methods of assessing exercise intensity had the advantage of being readily transferable to other physical activities performed outside the exercise class setting. Participants in both groups were given advice and guidance about performing additional forms of physical activity.

Participants were encouraged to attend two exercise classes per week, in addition to other physical activities of their choice. This allowed them to accumulate 30 minutes or more of moderate-intensity physical activity on most, preferably all, days of the week, which came within the current guidelines (American College of Sports Medicine 1990; Pate et al. 1995). Other physical activities included: London Central YMCA 'The complete pre- and postnatal fitness plan video' for home use (Gaskill 1992), aquanatal and other exercise classes, swimming, brisk walking and cycling (Pate et al. 1995). The exercise video for home use was 45–55 min in duration and followed the same format and design of the exercise class. The aquanatal classes in the local leisure centres were of 45 min in duration, with exercises in the water designed to take account of the physiological changes of pregnancy and the associated physiological effects of exercise in the water. Funding was available to reimburse participants with the admission cost of one physical activity per week at a leisure centre. Participants were recommended to contact the researcher to discuss other physical activity undertaken for inclusion in the programme.

# Psychological outcome measures

A number of psychological indicators were assessed during early pregnancy to measure baseline values and any changes over time. A questionnaire booklet was prepared to collect data, which included all outcome measures and additional information required for the study at each of the time points, i.e. early, late and after pregnancy (see Appendix 10).

### Psychological well-being questionnaire

Evidence linking physical activity with psychological well-being comes from a number of sources already discussed within the literature review. Mental health is one of the important components of complete well-being that has been associated with exercise. Physical activity may help people cope with stress more effectively and reduce emotional reactions to stressful life events.

One of the first issues to be considered for exercise studies was the selection of suitable measures of psychological experience. Many measures, such as questionnaires or interviews, are designed to assess psychopathophysiology. This may reveal scores that might warrant clinical attention and therefore their application to the general population may not be appropriate. Scores from the general population may initially be so low before training (floor effect) that there would be limited scope for further gains.

Outcome measures widely used in exercise studies such as the Profile of Mood States (POMS) developed by McNair et al. (1981) were better adapted for assessing *affect* in the general population. However, even these measures failed to capture the positive feelings of well-being that are experienced and reported by the general population, which were more than just the absence of anxiety or depression.

The outcome measurement tool chosen for this study was the psychological well-being questionnaire that was developed and validated by Moses et al. (1989). It was a 'self-report' questionnaire designed for use in a normal population. It consists of 36 items selected from the literature concerning responses to exercise, and is intended to assess perceptions of coping ability, feelings of mastery and subjective changes that accompanied exercise. Validity and reliability of 30 of the 36 items in the questionnaire had been previously confirmed by factor analysis performed on questionnaires completed by volunteers ($n = 102$). Three distinct factors emerged from this: perceptions of coping assets, i.e. perceived ability to cope; perceptions of coping deficits, i.e. perceived inability to cope; and perceptions of physical well-being. Perception of coping assets (14 items) predominantly contains positive coping statements and feelings about 'self' whereas the perception of coping deficits (10 items) consists of negative feelings and poor competence. Perception of physical well-being (six items) is concerned with perceived physical status. The internal reliability of the scales showed satisfactory levels of consistency across items and separate presentations of the questionnaire. Internal consistency was found to be satisfactory with the same participants ($n = 75$) on the two separate occasions. The remaining six items were excluded from the analysis during the validity and reliability studies (Moses et al. 1989).

The 30 items analysed in the validity and reliability studies by Moses et al. (1989) were incorporated into the present questionnaire. As each question was scaled on a 5-point scale (0–4), the perception of coping assets score could range between 0 and 56, with perception of coping deficits ranging between 0 and 40 and perception of physical well-being ranging between 0 and 24. Higher scores for perceived coping assets and perceived physical well-being reflected positive perceptions of both coping assets and physical well-being, whereas lower scores for perceived coping deficits signified a positive response in participants.

The psychological indicators of perceptions of coping assets and coping deficits encompass psychological and emotional factors contributing to perceptions in the ability to cope. Therefore, for the purpose of this present study, the three psychological indicators of well-being assessed by this questionnaire are identified as perceptions of coping assets (positive psychological well-being), perceptions of coping deficits (negative psychological well-being) and perceptions of physical well-being.

The 'self-report' questionnaire was designed for a normal population but had not been used during pregnancy. After consultation with the authors (Moses et al.), it was suggested that there was no reason why the questionnaire could not be used as a measurement tool for outcomes of psychological well-being with pregnant women.

**Maternal adjustments and attitudes questionnaire**

Kumar et al. (1984) developed this 'self-report' measurement tool which assessed the psychological condition of a woman during pregnancy, and the ways in which she views herself, her baby and those close to her. The background for the development of the questionnaire was the indication that pregnancy, especially the first pregnancy, was a watershed in a woman's life and childbirth was associated with increased risks of both psychotic and neurotic disturbance (Brockington et al. 1982; Kumar 1982; Kumar and Brockington 1988). There was also a suggestion that psychological stresses in pregnancy can adversely affect the physical health of both mother and baby (Erikson 1976).

The development and validation of the questionnaire were designed specifically to investigate patterns of change in the perceptions of maternal adjustment to pregnancy, attitudes to marital relationships and attitudes to the baby. The acronym MAMA refers to maternal adjustment and maternal attitudes.

Kumar et al. (1984) carried out the reliability of the 60-item questionnaire on first-time mothers (n = 119), with reliability being examined in two ways by test–retest and split-half reliability. Validity of the questionnaire was approached by comparing findings obtained by different methods, i.e. self-reported scoring of the somatic symptoms subgroup category compared with interview response on several symptoms, which was followed through with t-tests. Interview ratings of satisfaction with marital relationship were made on a 4-point scale and followed through with t-tests. This was repeated with three of the other four subgroup categories. Comparison with interview findings and questionnaire data provided good evidence for criterion validity. The two estimates of reliability were found to be reassuringly high and, taken together with the measure of criterion-related validity, suggested that women did not respond haphazardly and the questionnaire was actually measuring the subgroup categories.

Until reliability and validation of this questionnaire were undertaken, there had been some criticism of the use of self-rating questionnaires aimed at assessing marital relationships (Quinton et al. 1976) and self-assessment of sexual function (Bentler and Abramson 1981). However, the relevant scales of the MAMA questionnaire were found to meet these essential requirements. The questionnaire has been used widely in psychological research for the measurement of psychological well-being in studies during pregnancy (Green 1990a; Green et al. 1990).

Most women can complete the questionnaire without difficulty in less than 10 minutes. It was also found to be acceptable and interesting, and perceived as relevant to women (Kumar et al. 1984). There has been no attempt to disguise the purpose of the questions and the questionnaire does not contain a 'lie' score. There was random rotation of the rating scales (n = 30), which was intended to reduce 'response set'. The questionnaire specifically assesses perceptions of body image, perceptions of somatic symptoms, attitudes to marital relationships, attitudes to sex, and attitudes to pregnancy and the baby. Scores range from 1 to 4, with 1 classed as the 'most desirable' score and 4 the 'least desirable' score. However, for the purpose of the present study, scores obtained were presented in the opposite direction from the original questionnaire. This was intended to facilitate the demonstration of similar trends in either a negative or a positive direction when comparing the findings from these dependent indicators and other dependent indicators being investigated.

### Edinburgh Postnatal Depression Scale

The Edinburgh Postnatal Depression Scale (EPDS), derived from the earlier work of Snaith et al. (1978), was developed by Cox et al. (1987) as a screening instrument to detect depression among women in the early postpartum period. Its principal feature is the emphasis on psychological rather than somatic symptoms of depression. This avoids the possible confounding of psychological symptoms of depression with normal physiological functions associated with child-bearing. The measure was found to have satisfactory sensitivity and specificity in the detection of postnatal depression, when compared with diagnosis made by standardized interview (Cox et al. 1987; Harris et al. 1989). The measure has the benefit of being short with only 10 items; it has been found to be widely acceptable and easy to use by postnatal women in the community (Cox et al. 1987; Murray and Carothers 1990). As a result, the EPDS has become the measure of choice in studies of depression in child-bearing.

The measure has been satisfactorily validated as an assessment of the emotional well-being of women during the antenatal period (Hannah et al. 1990; Murray and Cox 1990; Green et al. 1991) and postnatal period (Harris et al. 1989; Murray and Carothers 1990). Therefore, the EPDS is a suitable tool for measurement of emotional well-being through pregnancy, the postpartum year and beyond (Kumar and Robson 1984). Its usefulness in estimating psychological well-being in the postnatal period was confirmed by Harris et al. (1989) who found the EPDS to be superior to other scales for measuring depression such as the Beck Inventory (Beck and Steer 1979).

Timing and frequency of administration of the EPDS, and the attitude and knowledge of the person administering the scale, are factors that need to be considered. Disadvantages identified may include: false-negative and -positive readings; stereotyping of individuals as already being 'depressed' when it was known that they had been required to repeat the questionnaire; and the potential ethical situation arising when there was doubt about the score obtained (Cox and Holden 1993). These issues were considered in relation to this present study and it was recommended, that it would be appropriate, in this study, to administer this 'once-only' questionnaire to women between 12 and 16 weeks in the postpartum period, to provide information on psychological well-being.

# Pregnancy and birth outcome measures

Numerous studies have investigated the effects of exercise during pregnancy on pregnancy and birth outcomes. In general, there is agreement that regular moderate exercise during pregnancy is safe for mother and baby (Huch and Erkkola 1990; Pivarnik 1998; Kramer 2000). There is inconclusive evidence to support any relationship that exercise during pregnancy can influence labour and delivery. There remains concern that exercise during pregnancy may cause a risk of preterm delivery, prolonged and difficult labour, fetal compromise and adverse effects on the newborn.

### Pregnancy and birth outcomes

Obstetric and medical conditions that developed during and after pregnancy were recorded in terms of minor and major complications. Any condition that could affect the health of mother or baby was categorized as a major complication, i.e. threatened abortion, antepartum haemorrhage, pre-eclampsia, hypertension and maternal infections. Minor disorders included the disorders of pregnancy and other minor conditions that did not affect the mother or pregnancy, e.g. mild nausea and vomiting, heartburn and constipation.

Delivery details included the following:

- Length of the gestation (weeks)
- Duration of labour (hours)
- Mode of delivery, i.e. normal spontaneous vertex delivery (SVD), instrumental delivery (forceps and Ventouse extraction) and surgical delivery (lower uterine segment caesarean section or LUSCS)
- Maternal complications experienced

Baby details included the following:

- Birthweight
- General condition of the baby at birth as assessed by Apgar score at 1 and 5 min
- Congenital or neonatal complications.

In the first instance, this factual information was obtained by postal questionnaire from the participants (see Appendix 12). This information was retrieved from the obstetric notes by the researcher when either the information was not directly available from the participants who had dropped out of the study or the information provided needed to have more detail.

## Recording physical activity

Physical activity is a complex behaviour, and patterns of activity fluctuate between and within individuals. It was extremely difficult to obtain reliable data about habitual levels of physical activity as a result of disagreement in the literature about what constitutes consistent levels of physical activity (Durnin 1992).

The subjective method of maintaining an activity diary is suggested to be the most pragmatic measure for monitoring physical activity (LaPorte et al. 1985). However, there have been few attempts to examine the validity and reliability of subjective methods (Lamb and Brodie 1991).

Activity diaries were included to enable episodes of physical activity to be recorded and monitored during the course of the study (see Appendix 11). This had the additional benefit of providing participants with the opportunity to record this information, which could then be summarized more accurately at each data-collection point. Participants in both groups were asked to describe physical activity undertaken in terms of when the activity was undertaken, the type of activity, and the duration and frequency (see Appendix 11). This information was requested at the three data-collection points, i.e. early pregnancy (12–16 weeks), late pregnancy (36–40 weeks) and after pregnancy (12–16 weeks). An attendance register was maintained at the exercise class for the participants in the intervention group, who could use this to give additional information of other physical activities undertaken (see Appendix 13).

This information was categorized into the following:

- Types of structured classes, e.g. aquanatal, aerobic, strength training, yoga classes
- Swimming
- Cycling
- Brisk walking
- Golf
- Badminton and tennis sessions
- Treadmill/Nordic skiing exercise
- Home exercise video.

Table 3.1 presents a summary of the information and questionnaires required at each time point of interest.

**Table 3.1** Timing of outcome measures

| | |
|---|---|
| *At recruitment:*<br>*8–12 weeks* | Personal details and activity levels in early pregnancy |
| *12–16 weeks* | **Psychological well-being questionnaire**<br>i.e. perceptions of coping assets (positive psychological well-being), coping deficits (negative psychological well-being) and physical well-being<br>**MAMA questionnaire**<br>i.e. perceptions of body image and somatic symptoms, and attitudes to marital relationships, sex and pregnancy<br>**Summary of physical activity and health status** |
| *36–40 weeks* | **Psychological well-being questionnaire**<br>i.e. perceptions of coping assets (positive psychological well-being), coping deficits (negative psychological well-being) and physical well-being<br>**MAMA questionnaire**<br>i.e. perceptions of body image and somatic symptoms, and attitudes to marital relationships, sex and pregnancy<br>**Summary of physical activity/health status** |
| *12–16 weeks* | **Psychological well-being questionnaire**<br>i.e. perceptions of coping assets (positive psychological well-being), coping deficits (negative psychological well-being) and physical well-being<br>**MAMA questionnaire**<br>i.e. perceptions of body image and somatic symptoms, and attitudes to marital relationships, sex and baby<br>**Edinburgh Postnatal Depression Scale**<br>i.e. emotional well-being and depression<br>**Summary of physical activity/health status**<br>**Summary of pregnancy/birth outcomes**<br>i.e. length of gestation, duration of labour, method of delivery, Apgar score at 1 and 5 min after birth, birth-weight, and any maternal or neonatal complications |
| *On completion* | **Total number of physical activities**, i.e. from 12–16 weeks of pregnancy until 12–16 weeks after delivery |

## Follow-up of outcome measures and retention of participants

The initial questionnaire in early pregnancy was enclosed within the information pack given at the time of recruitment. If this was not returned, a second questionnaire was posted out with an accompanying information letter about the study (see Appendix 10). This letter gave a reminder of the study and informed the participants that postal questionnaires would continue to be sent to their home address at the appropriate data-collection points unless they contacted the researcher. A poster giving details of the exercise class was enclosed for those participants allocated to the intervention group who did not return questionnaires or who did not attend the exercise class. Postal questionnaires were issued to all participants within the 2-week period before the data-collection time point. Questionnaires were re-issued 3 weeks later if the original questionnaire was not returned.

Three postnatal reunions at the maternity hospital were organized during the course of the study. This was an informal gathering of all participants in the study and their new babies. Invitations were sent out to participants in both groups who had delivered their babies and remained in the study.

## Controlling threats to validity

Threats to the validity of the research study consisted of two types: internal validity related to the experiment itself and external validity related to generalization of the results to other situations (Rees 1997). These issues were given careful consideration in the planning of this present study to reduce the threats to validity of the research design.

Random selection had been identified as the key to controlling threats to external validity. Randomization of participants to groups allowed the assumption that they were equivalent at the beginning of the research. This design controlled for history and testing which occurred equally with the maturation of groups (Thomas and Nelson 1990). This allowed control of the sources of invalidity based on non-equivalency of groups, which included selection biases and selection maturation interaction. The inclusion of only first-time prospective mothers as participants and the introduction of a control group reduced any confounding bias. The validity and reliability of the outcome measures for the dependent indicators have been previously discussed.

A potentially confounding variable was the 'expectation effect' of the participants knowing that they were in a research study and being aware of the effort and time spent with them. Jamieson and Flood (1993) have suggested that few experiments paid sufficient attention to this particular issue of the 'expectation effect'. This was an important factor to consider from the point of view of the research design in relation to the participants in the control and intervention groups. As the main researcher, I tried to ensure that the intervention was the only difference between the two groups.

The intervention was not an artificial setting but was a structured exercise programme in all respects, i.e. designed exercise programme, exercise hall and qualified instructor. The potentially confounding variable introduced by between-instructor variability was avoided by having one instructor present at all classes. This factor, in itself, could have introduced the confounding variable of experimenter bias towards the intervention group.

Retaining participants within the study was of concern especially because of the duration of the participation. In general, it is common for participants to drop out of randomized controlled trials of exercise interventions (Ward and Morgan 1984). This is mainly because participants do not wish to exercise in the first place. A drop-out rate of 20% has been reported in controlled trials, with some exercise studies having a drop-out rate as high as 40–50% (Ward and Morgan 1984). It has been argued that 80–85% is the maximum possible retention in exercise studies, even in populations with good facilities and positive attitudes to exercise. Steptoe (1992) suggests that the crucial problem for controlled trials of psychological response is not so much that drop-out should be minimized, but that drop-out should not be selective across experimental conditions. Thomas and Nelson (1990) state that any type of experimental design cannot control the retention of participants. They suggest that these problems can be handled in advance of the research by carefully explaining the research to the participants and the need for them to carry it through and complete the study.

## Data management

All participants were given a unique code number which was used when handling data. Responses to information obtained from questionnaires and notes were entered into the database appropriately coded. Data for participants were stored in the computer database using participant's code numbers (Department of Health 1994, 1998).

## Data analysis

Statistical analyses were carried out using 'Minitab' statistics software package, which is essentially a package for data exploration and data manipulation.

Repeated measure analyses of variances (ANOVAs) were carried out to investigate differences between the two groups (i.e. exercise and control groups) at the three time points (i.e. early, late and after pregnancy). The Minitab GLM (General Linear Model) command was used to carry out the repeated measure ANOVAs. The time points of interest were: early pregnancy (12–16 weeks), late pregnancy (36–40 weeks) and after pregnancy (12–16 weeks). Significance level used was $p < 0.05$. It is recognised that there is a risk of increased type 1 errors, with the number of comparisons that were being conducted. Some protection against this increased risk was available from the use of the multiple-comparison test.

A follow-up multiple-comparison procedure with a simultaneous 95% confidence level was undertaken if a significant *interaction* of intervention group/time was indicated. This follow-up procedure allowed further, more detailed investigation of any differences between the groups for each of the outcome indicators in the amount of change reported from early pregnancy (12–16 weeks) to late pregnancy (36–40 weeks), early pregnancy (12–16 weeks) to after pregnancy (12–16 weeks), and late pregnancy (36–40 weeks) to after pregnancy (12–16 weeks).

Repeated measure ANOVAs were undertaken with the following outcome indicators:

- Perceptions of coping assets (positive psychological well-being)
- Perceptions of coping deficits (negative psychological well-being)
- Perceptions of physical well-being
- Perceptions of body image
- Perceptions of somatic symptoms
- Attitudes to marital relationships
- Attitudes to sex
- Attitudes to pregnancy and the baby.

The assumptions of the repeated measures ANOVAs were assessed by means of the tests of sphericity and residual and probability plots. All of the indicators considered in the analysis showed no evidence against any of the assumptions using these approaches.

Two-sample $t$-tests were also undertaken between the two groups (i.e. exercise and control), with each of the above outcome indicators in early pregnancy. This allowed baseline comparisons of each of the outcome indicators between the two groups before the intervention began.

Two-sample $t$-tests were undertaken to compare the groups in relation to the following outcome indicators measured on one occasion:

- Birthweight
- Episodes of physical activity.

The non-parametric chi-squared test allows comparison of the proportion of participants from research groups who fall into varying categories. Chi-squared tests were undertaken to investigate any differences between the control and intervention groups in terms of the following:

- Postnatal emotional well-being and depression
- Length of gestation (weeks)
- Duration of labour (hours)
- Apgar score of the baby at 1 and 5 min after birth
- Modes of delivery of the baby in each of the three categories of modes of delivery, i.e. normal (SVD), instrumental and surgical deliveries
- Physical activity levels reported in early pregnancy in each of the four categories, i.e. inactive, occasionally active, regularly active and very active
- Drop-out rate of participants during the study.

Correlation analyses were undertaken after pregnancy using Pearson's product–moment coefficient of correlations. This analysis was conducted to determine whether there was any relationship between the frequency of total activity and the responses of the three psychological indicators of coping assets (positive psychological well-being), coping deficits (negative psychological well-being) and physical well-being after pregnancy.

Descriptive statistics were used to present the following findings:

- Line graphs illustrated any patterns of change in the outcome indicators during and after pregnancy
- Bar graph demonstrated the frequency in the modes of delivery
- Frequency distribution of total activity for the control and intervention groups.

Tables indicated relevant information related to the following:

- Demographic details of participants
- Participants in the study
- Mode of delivery
- Maternal complications
- Frequency and distribution of the types of physical activity undertaken during the study.

In summary, this section has provided detailed information of the methods and research design used within the present study. The next two sections provide additional information to the reader as mentioned at the start of the chapter.

# Pilot study

The pilot study was undertaken as a preparatory measure to test the methodology before commencing the main study. This section is included because it was an essential prerequisite to the overall research design for the main study. At the time, I was aware of the need to test out the methodology, but it was only on hindsight that the true worth of this stage was appreciated. I was eager to commence and proceed with the main study because it was expected to be at least 2 years in duration.

It is hoped that those readers who are new to research will take time to read this section. I hope that it will emphasize to them the value of detailed preparation and evaluation to provide an efficient and effective research design, and avoid any unnecessary practical and operational problems likely to be encountered.

The design of the pilot study was restricted by the initial limitations stipulated by hospital management and the resources available. Ethical approval was obtained from the local health board. The overall aim of the pilot study was to evaluate and assess the proposed methodology in terms of the following four main areas of interest:

1. Efficiency and effectiveness of the recruitment procedure
2. Exercise programme in relation to the timing of the sessions, the venue and the content of the programme
3. Data-collection tools, collation, analysis and storage of data, and relevance and value of the data obtained
4. Resources.

The pilot study was a two-group, randomized, controlled research design. The control group continued with the existing antenatal preparation of parents for pregnancy, childbirth and the transition to parenthood. In addition, the intervention group participated in a structured antenatal and postnatal exercise programme.

All the information obtained from the pilot study was evaluated and assessed to ensure that the final methodology would be efficient and appropriate to meet the aims of the main study. Evaluation included the researcher conducting a semi-structured interview with the participants and health professionals involved in the study, to gain subjective views and constructive feedback about all aspects of the study. The data tools, data collation, analysis and storage were reviewed in conjunction with the statistician and research supervisors. Each of these areas of interest is discussed separately

## Recruitment procedure

The following was the aim:

- To review and assess both the efficiency and the effectiveness of the recruitment process. This was to ensure that the recruitment process encompassed all eligible women at their antenatal appointment, to provide the opportunity for them to participate in the study.
- To determine the number of women eligible for the study, the number of women who agreed to participate in the study and the number of participants who continued with and/or completed the study.
- To evaluate the consent and information forms and the recruitment procedures through discussion with the antenatal women and all health professionals involved in the study.
- Hospital management had previously agreed to the study with the following stipulations being made: women were to be recruited to the study during the first antenatal appointment at the selected clinic. All contact about the research study was to be conducted through the medical clerkess in the reception area. Midwifery clinic staff were not to be involved in recruitment to the study. Women who agreed to participate in the study would be asked to remain after their appointment to meet with the researcher for further information.

Participants to be recruited were healthy women during their first pregnancy. The researcher identified first-time prospective mothers on the clinic appointment list before the clinic started. The medical records clerkess issued an initial recruitment letter to these women on arrival for their appointment. This letter was to be returned to the appointment desk and then forwarded to the researcher, to arrange consent from the consultant obstetrician, where applicable.

Immediately after their appointment at the clinic (lasting about 2 hours), the participants had to meet with the researcher. During this meeting, they were given information about their code number, group allocation and further information related to the group. Consent forms were signed, information was given to the participants about the study and further arrangements were made about collecting the data.

Participants were recruited during each of the first three of five time periods of interest when data were collected:

1. Early pregnancy (12–16 weeks)
2. Mid-pregnancy (24–28 weeks)

3. Late pregnancy (36–40 weeks)
4. Birth to 4 weeks after birth
5. After pregnancy (12–16 weeks).

Once recruited, participants remained in the pilot for at least two data-collection points. This allowed a snapshot picture only between two time points, to enable the study to be completed in a shorter time span, i.e. between 8 and 10 months.

## Recruitment procedure and findings

### Details of the groups (n = 22)

The number of women eligible for recruitment was 25, i.e. control group (n = 13) and intervention group (n = 12). Three women allocated to the control group declined to participate in the study and a total of 10 participants was recruited to the control group. Table 3.2 presents the recruitment and retention of participants within the pilot study.

A total of 12 participants was recruited to the intervention group. Of these, six did not attend any exercise classes, i.e. 50%. A further participant attended one class only. The exercise class was regularly attended by the remaining five participants, i.e. 42% of the total recruited (12) and 83% of the participants (6) who attended the exercise classes.

**Table 3.2** Recruitment and retention of participants in the pilot study

| Subjects | Number | % |
| --- | --- | --- |
| Women eligible for the study | 77 | |
| Women who agreed to participate | 39 | 100 |
| Participants who remained to meet with the researcher, i.e. control (n = 13); intervention (n = 12) | 25 | 64 |
| Participants recruited to control group (three declined) | 10 | 100 |
| Participants recruited to the intervention group | 12 | 100 |
| Participants who failed to meet with the researcher | 14 | 36 |
| Participants who completed the study (control group) | 8 | 80 |
| Participants who completed the study (intervention group) | 6 | 50 |

### Evaluation of the study

This was in the form of a semi-structured interview. It was mainly conducted by telephone with the participants in the control group and either by telephone or 'face-to-face' interview with participants in the intervention group.

From evaluation of the recruitment process, most of the participants agreed that time was restricted at the clinic. This was because of the length of the appointment itself, and other considerations such as family members who had already been waiting for a few hours and transport arrangements. Participants indicated that it would be more convenient if the study had been discussed as part of their appointment in the clinic. It was also felt to be a disadvantage that the clinic staff 'knew nothing at all' about the study. Both the participants and the clinic staff suggested that it would be helpful if an information leaflet had been available to participants and staff at the time of recruitment. This need was reinforced when several pregnant women were given inaccurate information about the study by the midwifery staff.

Staff evaluation of the recruitment process indicated that it would improve efficiency if the midwifery staff were involved in the recruitment process. Medical records staffs did not report any problems with their involvement with the study and were satisfied to continue. However, they stipulated that medical notes had to remain in the medical records department.

No problems were found with any of the consent forms by any health professionals. However, two participants objected to their general practitioner/midwife being notified of their participation in the study. They felt that they would possibly be discouraged from attending the exercise class by the health professionals.

Recruitment for the study was found to be slow, considering the number of women who were eligible for the study from the clinic appointment list. It was found that either many women were not being offered the opportunity to participate in the study or the obstetrician was not being asked to give consent for the woman to participate in the study.

Basically, the restrictions placed on the methodology by hospital management had contributed to an inefficient and inconvenient system of recruitment and data collection for both participants and staff involved in the study.

The findings from the pilot study were presented to hospital management and suggestions were made to improve the methodology. These amendments were agreed and their implementation was given full support.

**Proposed amendments to recruitment procedure**

- Recruitment would take place at all the available antenatal clinics to ensure prompt recruitment of numbers for the main study.

- Midwives at the clinic would now be involved with the recruit-ment process in terms of gaining consent from participants, gaining consent from the consultant obstetrician and giving the participants the sealed and coded information pack. An equal number of information packs were made up for both groups before the main study commenced. These packs were sealed and allocated a code number on the outside of the envelope. The clinic staff were not aware of the allocated group. The researcher was the only person who knew this. Packs were available in the clinic for staff for distribution to the participants at the time of gaining consent from them. The clinic staff then forwarded details of participants and the code number on the information pack to the researcher. These amendments would remove further meeting with the researcher after this appointment, allow the participants to be allocated to their group at this time and also enable them to complete the initial information during this appointment time.
- Participants would be followed up within 1 week of recruitment by a telephone call from the researcher, to give them the oppor-tunity to discuss the study further, if required.
- All staff involved with the study would be invited to attend a presentation of the study, to discuss the importance of the recruitment of eligible participants and the extent of the health professionals' role in the process.
- Information letters to general practitioners/midwives were avail-able but would be issued only at the woman's request.

### Exercise programme

The exercise programme was designed to consider the physiological changes of pregnancy. It was based on the London Central YMCA (1992) programme for exercise during and after pregnancy. This programme is endorsed by the Royal College of Midwives and complies with the ACOG's guidelines for exercise during pregnancy (cited in Artal Mittlemark et al. 1991a). The aim was:

- To review the content/timing/convenience/venue of classes
- To evaluate subjective opinion of the exercise classes, 'self-instruct' home tapes and exercise leaflets
- To evaluate adherence to the exercise class sessions and the home exercise programme.

Participants allocated to the intervention group were advised to attend three structured exercise classes per week provided within the maternity hospital venue. This would allow participants to meet the current recommendations for physical activity, i.e. adults should accumulate 30 minutes or more of moderate-intensity physical activity on most, preferably all, days of the week (American College of Sports Medicine 1990; Pate et al. 1995).

The exercise class was offered at a variety of venues and times during the day and evening. Participants were given instruction about how to take their own pulse rate during the exercise class. This was followed with practice sessions and an instruction leaflet for home use. An audiocassette tape and audiovisual tape of the exercise programme were available for home use.

## Evaluation of the exercise programme

The preferred time for the structured exercise class was in the early evening between 6 and 7pm. The participants felt that this time was more convenient if they were working and attending evening parenthood education classes. The general recreation hall in the hospital was the venue of choice because it was conveniently placed with easy access to and availability of toilet and changing facilities.

Evaluation of the exercise class was satisfactory in relation to content, duration and organization. However, some of the participants found it awkward to record their own pulse rate during the class. None of the participants reported using the audiocassettes of exercise programmes, but exercise videocassettes were found to be useful. Postnatal participants preferred to bring their baby to the class, because it was difficult for them to arrange babysitters.

Attending three exercise classes per week proved to be difficult for participants to achieve. All participants attended one exercise class per week and two exercise classes on a few occasions. They did report participation or attendance at other physical activities that they wished to continue because it suited their social lifestyle. This was reviewed and discussed at length with research supervisors. It was decided to encourage participants to attend two structured exercise classes per week, but to extend the study to include a variety of other agreed physical activities, such as aquanatal classes and swimming, brisk walking and golf (Pate et al. 1995). This incorporated a flexible approach to meet the needs of the participants.

Participants in both groups maintained a diary of physical activity. This allowed the total number of physical activities to be recorded over the course of the study. It also enabled them to summarize accurately their average weekly episodes of physical activity required at each data-collection point.

**Adherence and drop-out**

Participants did not want to come to the class alone and felt that it would be an advantage initially to bring along a friend. Also, most participants wanted only to attend the exercise class once or twice a week. Three times a week was impossible for many participants because of other activities attended and parenthood education classes.

Many participants currently attended the aquanatal classes provided in conjunction with the maternity unit and leisure centres in Ayrshire. One woman reported that she had 'dropped out' of the study because she had been apprehensive about locating her pulse rate and had only guessed it.

Participants felt that it would have been easy to drop out of the study after they had missed one or two exercise classes. They felt obliged to return because it was important to the study.

**Control group**

In general, the control participants felt that they should either not be exercising at all or be restricted as to what exercise they were allowed to undertake. They also felt that they were just guessing about whether they were regular or occasional exercisers, because they could not remember the number of times that they had exercised.

Control participants felt that there was so much information required by different people during pregnancy that, by the time they had received the questionnaires, they had forgotten the reason for the study. This made them averse to completing the questionnaire until the reminder phone call prompted them to do so.

**Proposed amendments to the exercise programme**

- Classes would now be offered twice a week between 6 and 7pm in the General Recreation Hall at Ayrshire Central Hospital.
- Pulse rates would still be located and recorded during the exercise class but, in addition, the 'Borg's Perceived Rating of Exertion Scale' (RPE) would be available for those participants who were initially finding difficulty in locating and recording their pulse rates. Information leaflets on locating and recording pulse rates and the use of 'RPE' scales would be available for participants to use at other exercise sessions.
- Participants were welcome to bring along a friend if numbers permitted, and a midwife friend would be available at the classes to take care of any babies who attended with their mothers.

- Exercise videos (YMCA 'Antenatal and Postnatal Exercise Programme') would continue to be available for loan by individual participants.
- Other physical activities could now be included within the exercise programme to enable participants to meet their weekly 'exercise' requirements satisfactorily. These activities included: other exercise classes such as aerobics or aquanatal classes at local leisure centres, swimming, cycling, golf, brisk walking, etc.
- A class register would be introduced with a section for other physical activities to be included for use by participants attending the exercise class.
- A poster about the intervention group would be sent out at regular intervals to those who did not attend the class for 2 or 3 weeks without any contact.
- Participants in the 'control' group would be reassured that they could continue with their usual lifestyle in terms of physical activity.
- Participants in both groups would incorporate an activity diary within the study to enable an accurate summary of physical activity at the data-collection points. The activity diary would be amended to aid completion and this information would be collected as the study progressed. These amendments were made for convenience to the participants and to provide a total for the number of additional classes attended during the course of the study

**Data-collection tools**

The aim was the following:

1. To review/evaluate the questionnaires in relation to the:
   - response rate
   - time taken to complete questionnaires
   - subjective views of questionnaires/other data-collection tools
   - distribution and retrieval process for questionnaires.
2. To review/evaluate the pregnancy and birth outcomes in relation to the:
   - method of data collection during this stage
   - method of coding participants, data collection, storage and retrieval
   - appropriateness of the data collection
   - method and efficiency of monitoring progress of pregnancy and the information regarding any problems arising.

3. To review method of collating information in relation to physical activity.

The following questionnaires were completed at the time points of interest:

- Well-being questionnaire
- Maternal attitude and adaptation to pregnancy
- Trait–State Inventory
- Edinburgh Postnatal Depression Scale (postnatal only)
- Pregnancy details
- Pregnancy and birth outcomes (postnatal only)
- Activity details
- Evaluation of data collation, analysis and storage.

All participants ($n = 6$) in the intervention group completed the required questionnaires. In the control group eight of the ten participants completed the questionnaires. All felt that these questionnaires were too long and sometimes they were unsure of what was required in the response to the questions. There was also considerable delay in returning questionnaires and many were returned incomplete.

Gaining information from medical/obstetric notes proved to be difficult because these notes were usually being used elsewhere by other health professionals. The retrieval process was satisfactory for data, which was coded and stored in the computer database.

Data-collection tools were found to be time-consuming to complete and issued too frequently. This contributed to poor response rate and return of incomplete information. Evaluation of data collated was undertaken in conjunction with the statistician. This resulted in a reduction in the number of data-collection points to the three time points identified as being essential to gain meaningful information, i.e. early pregnancy (12–16 weeks), late pregnancy (36–40 weeks) and after pregnancy (12–16 weeks). Information was removed that was identified as being irrelevant or superfluous to the study aims. Subsequently, a 'user-friendly' booklet of questionnaires was designed to collect all relevant information.

### Amendments to data handling

- Information obtained was reviewed for relevancy within the context of the study. It was felt that the responses to the Trait–State Inventory was of little value and this was removed. Other information deemed irrelevant to the present study was subsequently removed, e.g. perceptions of labour and delivery.

- A booklet of questionnaires was designed to incorporate all the information necessary. This included a summary of relevant information about health and labour/delivery details. Medical notes would be required only in the event of missing data or details that needed further investigation.
- A letter reminding participants about the study was included with the issue of each questionnaire booklet. The first questionnaire would be included within the information pack. Thereafter, subsequent questionnaires would be posted to the home address 1 week before the time range for data collection. A second questionnaire would be posted out 2 weeks within the 4-week range. Stamped addressed envelopes were included. In addition, the participants could also give completed questionnaires to their midwife or other health professional for postage through the internal mailing system.

Results were discussed with both the statistician and research supervisors. It was decided that the three time points identified as obtaining valuable information were to be retained, i.e. early (12–16 weeks) pregnancy, late (36–40 weeks) pregnancy and after (12–16 weeks) pregnancy. There was poor response to the questionnaires issued during the second trimester and at delivery, with most information being omitted or incomplete. These data-collection points did not reveal any informative data and were omitted from the main study. It was decided to rotate the direction of the responses in the original MAMA questionnaire because this would ensure consistency in the direction of positive and negative responses from all questionnaires. The sample size for the main study was calculated based on current results.

The sample size for the main study was estimated using the variables of perceptions of body image and coping assets (positive psychological well-being) to determine the overall sample size necessary to gain statistical significance. From the findings, assumptions were made indicating that the study would require a minimum of 30 participants in each of the two groups to complete the study for a power of 0.90. Based on these calculations, it was recommended to recruit at least 50 participants into each group once the drop-out rate from the pilot study was considered.

Statistical tests would include repeated measure ANOVAs to determine whether there were any differences between the two groups over time for each of the psychological variables. Follow-up multiple-comparison tests with a simultaneous 95% confidence level would be undertaken when any significant differences were indicated. Two-sample $t$-tests would be undertaken with those dependent variables measured once during the study, e.g. length of gestation, duration of pregnancy, Apgar scores, birthweight and postnatal emotional well-being. Chi-squared tests would determine whether there were any differences in the mode of delivery of the baby and exercise levels in early pregnancy.

## Resources

The resources required for the study were reviewed. It was agreed that funding would enable essential resources for the study. Application for funding was agreed by:

1. North Ayrshire and Arran NHS Trust Lottery Committee to purchase a music system for the large hall, floor mats and exercise videos.
2. Ayrshire and Arran Health Board provided funding to reimburse the participants with the admission fee for one activity per week at the leisure centre of their choice for the duration of the study.

### Summary of the pilot study

The pilot study proved to be more worthwhile and valuable than the researcher had anticipated. Findings from the pilot study made a significant contribution to the final research design for the main study. A summary of these amendments included: a more efficient process for the recruitment of participants; the removal of irrelevant data and reduction in the number of data-collection points; and the design of an 'easy-to-use' questionnaire booklet for data collection. The structured exercise class would be scheduled at a convenient time and venue for women and babies could accompany mothers in the postnatal period. Additional activities were incorporated within the programme and an activity diary that was easy to complete was available for both groups of participants.

This section provided additional information about the preparation and planning for the research design used in the main study.

# Antenatal and postnatal exercise programmes

Pregnancy is distinguished by psychological and physiological changes and these have been detailed previously (see Chapter 2). The physiological changes are necessary to provide an optimal environment for the developing fetus and to maintain normal function for the mother. Many pregnant women often choose to exercise during pregnancy and after childbirth. These are very special times in a woman's life when extra care and caution during exercise are required.

Considered separately, pregnancy and exercise both have a complex interaction on the body systems. The impact that exercise may have on pregnancy gives cause for concern, especially with the body systems that they share. These include the cardiovascular, respiratory, metabolic and musculoskeletal systems. All forms of exercise undertaken during and after pregnancy need to be safe for the woman, her pregnancy and her baby.

The aim of this section is to provide the reader with more detailed information about the exercise programmes for pregnancy and after birth. The components of the exercise programme are detailed as well as specific considerations related to anatomical and physiological changes. Precautions, contraindications and guidelines for exercise during and after pregnancy are presented.

The overall purpose of the exercise programme was to maintain physical fitness and to prepare the body to cope with pregnancy, childbirth and the transition to parenthood. The design of the exercise programme followed sound ergonomic principles. It considered the anatomical, physiological and structural changes of pregnancy and the possible impact of exercise on these changes.

# Factors to be considered

1. The effects of the hormone relaxin on the body's connective and fibrous tissue, particularly in the ligaments of the joints and pelvic floor. This results in connective tissue laxity and joint instability, which continues until about 6 months after birth of the baby. The joints remain more susceptible to injury during the postnatal period.
2. The weakening of the abdominal muscles and any possible diastasis (separation).
3. Postural changes and changes in the centre of gravity as pregnancy progresses.
4. Cardiovascular changes.

The choice of appropriate exercise and the teaching of correct exercise technique are paramount. Exercise should be directed more towards the development of good posture, improved body awareness and control of movement than the development of the specific components of fitness.

**Warm-up**

*Aims*

- Take the joints through the full range of movements

- Become familiar with and introduce the mind to the sensations of movement and body
- Increase circulation and prepare the cardiovascular system by very low repetitive work; this allows the heart rate gradually to increase with exercise and provide the working muscles with adequate blood supply
- Prepare the neuromuscular response pattern
- Give the body time to prepare for more activity later
- Warm muscle groups to a temperature for optimum performance during the exercise programme.

All movements should be controlled. The warm-up includes exercises that increase the activity of the heart and circulatory system, joint mobility, posture and stretching exercises. Pregnant women 'warm up' quicker than when they were not pregnant. This is because of the increased cardiac output and circulating blood. However, more time is required during this period to prepare women for exercise, teaching points, posture and balance as pregnancy progresses.

Stretching of the muscles after the warm-up should be undertaken to promote relaxation and reduce tension. Stretches should be static.

## Aerobic component

*Aims*

- To improve and/or maintain aerobic capacity
- To increase body awareness and movement control.

## Muscular strength and endurance

*Aims*

- To make main muscle groups strong enough to support the skeletal structure and to maintain posture and body shape.
- Posture alters during pregnancy to compensate for the expanding abdomen. As a result, the pelvis often tips forward, causing an excessive curve in the lumbar spine. This leads to the baby protruding in front of the mother, with resultant distribution of weight, stressing the vulnerable areas of the lower back. Correction of this requires good use of the abdominal muscles and can also provide an excellent toning exercise to help regain a flat stomach after the birth. Women are encouraged to tilt their pelvis backwards, so that the baby is tucked in towards them and held securely by firm abdominal muscles. This stabilizes the lower back for the lumbar spine.

- To improve muscular endurance to aid good posture, reduce the risk of strain to the back and prepare for postpartum recovery.
- To promote muscle fitness, to enhance the woman's ability to cope with the demands of pregnancy.
- To maintain and develop muscle tone to increase self-confidence.

**Stretching**

*Aims*

- To reduce muscle tension and make the body feel more relaxed
- To maintain the range of movement of joints and muscles so that the body can work more efficiently
- To improve exercise technique by extending the range of body movement
- To maintain mobility rather than improve flexibility.

Stretching exercises are valuable for women during pregnancy for the reasons described above. However, all stretching exercises are carried out with care and supervision. Stretching should not be taken to the point of maximum resistance. Developmental stretching is contraindicated because this may overstretch ligaments already softened by hormonal action and may reduce the stability of the joints. Muscles should be stretched to counteract muscle cramping or muscle soreness and to relax the lower back.

**Cool down**

*Aims*

- To return the body gradually to the non-exercising state
- To relax in order to reduce physical tension
- To assist the body in the removal of substances that may contribute to muscle soreness
- To assist the venous return of blood to the heart, to prevent pooling of blood in the lower body.

*Precautions*

Exercise in the supine position is contraindicated after the fourth month of pregnancy. Blood flow from the lower body is returned to the heart by the main blood vessel called the inferior vena cava. The weight of the growing fetus may occlude this flow and result in the woman feeling light-headed and dizzy. Alternative safe positions should be suggested for exercise.

Joints are more relaxed during pregnancy and there is a greater level of flexibility. This renders women more susceptible to injury. Therefore, movements should be slow and controlled in order to facilitate good teaching and the opportunity to correct faulty positions as they occur.

- Avoid overstretching and overextending joints. Support joints as pregnancy advances.
- Avoid complicated movements, jerky movements and those that require any quick changes in direction.
- Design the programme to enable women easily to adopt one of several alternative ways to perform the individual exercises. These may be required as pregnancy advances.

## Considerations for the postnatal period

Women are not recommended to join an exercise class before the postnatal examination has been undertaken around 6 weeks after the birth of the baby. Before this period, women should continue with the gentle exercises routinely given by the obstetric physiotherapist.

Floor abdominal exercises should not be commenced until it has been confirmed that there is no separation of the abdominal muscles. The separation of the recti abdominis sheath and stretching of the linea alba occurs during all pregnancies, to some degree. This normally reduces after birth, provided that the muscles are not weakened or overstretched. Abdominal muscles are unable to work efficiently if there is separation of the recti abdominis sheath. In severe cases, the linea alba splits during pregnancy and diastasis recti abdominis may persist into the postnatal period. An appropriate qualified individual (e.g. exercise instructor, obstetric physiotherapist or health professional) should check for diastasis recti abdominis before postnatal exercises are undertaken, especially those involving abdominal muscles. On assessment, one to two fingerbreadths (maximum) between the abdominal rectus sheath of muscles is normal and acceptable to allow gentle introduction to abdominal floor exercise.

For at least 6 months *avoid*: sit ups and stomach crunches (longer if there is separation of abdominal muscles) and lifting both legs with legs straight. *The pelvic floor requires special consideration.* The muscles of the pelvic floor are slightly toned by general exercise but specific pelvic floor exercises are vital both during and after pregnancy. These will tone the muscles to avoid the common problems associated with pelvic floor problems in the postnatal period.

# Guidelines for exercise during pregnancy

Guidelines for exercise during pregnancy were first introduced by the American College of Obstetricians and Gynecologists (ACOG) in 1985 (Artal Mittlemark et al. 1991c). These were developed in response to a growing number of requests from women and health professionals who wanted information in this area. The initial guidelines were controversial because they were thought to be too specific to be general guidelines for exercise during pregnancy (Gauthier 1986). However, these guidelines were intended only to be used with the 'commonsense' approach and did not prevent women from adopting a more individualized approach to exercise. These detailed guidelines were then replaced by less conservative guidelines in 1994 (ACOG 1994). The revised guidelines acknowledge evidence that indicated that healthy women with normal pregnancies may safely engage in many types of exercise. This does not compromise the health of the fetus or complicate the pregnancy, labour or delivery (Sternfield 1997).

The previous guidelines are summarized within this section because these were followed during the present study. In addition, the more recent guidelines are also included to give the reader up to date information.

### ACOG guidelines 1985 (cited in Artal Mittlemark et al. 1991c)

*Pregnancy and postpartum*

1. Regular exercise (at least three times a week) is preferable to intermittent activity.
2. Vigorous exercise should not be performed in hot, humid weather or during a period of febrile illness.
3. Ballistic movements (jerky, bouncy motions) should be avoided.
4. Deep flexion or extension of joints should be avoided because of connective tissue laxity. Activities that require jumping, jarring motions or rapid changes in direction should be avoided because of joint instability.
5. Vigorous exercise should be preceded by a 5-minute warm up. This can be accomplished by slow walking or stationary cycling with low resistance.
6. Vigorous exercise should be followed by a period of gradually declining activity that includes gentle stationary stretching. Connective tissue laxity increases the risk of joint injury, so stretches should not be taken to the point of maximum resistance.
7. Heart rate should be measured at times of peak activity. Target heart

rates and limits established in consultation with the physician should not be exceeded.

8. Care should be taken to rise gradually from the floor to avoid orthostatic hypotension. Some form of activity involving the legs should be continued for a brief period.

9. Liquids should be taken liberally before and after exercise to prevent dehydration. If necessary, activity should be interrupted to replenish fluids.

10. Women who have led sedentary lifestyles should begin with physical activity of very low intensity and advance activity levels very gradually.

### *Pregnancy only*

- Maternal heart rate should not exceed 140 beats/min.
- Strenuous exercise should not exceed 15 min in duration.
- No exercise should be performed in the supine position after the fourth month of gestation is complete.
- Exercises that employ the Valsalva manoeuvre should be avoided.
- Caloric intake should be adequate to meet not only the extra energy needs of pregnancy, but also of the exercises performed.
- Maternal core temperature should not exceed 38°C.

Note: activity should be stopped and a physician consulted if any unusual symptoms appear.

**Table 3.3** Heart rate guidelines for postpartum exercise

| Age (years) | Limit (beats/min)[a] | Maximum (beats/min) |
|---|---|---|
| 20 | 150 | 200 |
| 25 | 146 | 195 |
| 30 | 142 | 190 |
| 35 | 138 | 185 |
| 40 | 135 | 180 |
| 45 | 131 | 175 |

[a]Each figure represents 75% of the maximum heart rate that would be predicted for the corresponding age groups. Under proper medical supervision, more strenuous activity and higher heart rates may be appropriate.

### Exercise contraindications

The following includes conditions that should be considered contraindications to exercise during pregnancy:

- Pregnancy-induced hypertension
- Pre-term rupture of membranes
- Pre-term labour during previous or current pregnancy or both
- Incompetent cervix
- Persistent second- or third-stage bleeding
- Intrauterine growth retardation.

In addition, women with certain other medical or obstetric conditions, including chronic hypertension or active thyroid, cardiac, vascular or pulmonary disease, should be evaluated carefully in order to determine whether an exercise programme is appropriate.

Advice and guidance offered to women who want to exercise during and after pregnancy:

- Women who are starting exercise during pregnancy should begin at a very low intensity of exercise and gradually increase activity levels.
- Women already exercising can continue their existing programme and should amend exercise levels as pregnancy progresses.

### Avoid

- Performing in hot, humid weather or during a period of febrile illness.
- Activities that require jumping, jarring and ballistic movements (jerky, bouncy motions) or rapid changes in direction because of joint instability.
- Deep flexion or extension of joints because of connective tissue laxity.

### Warning signs

Pregnant women should be alerted to warning signs that should prompt them to stop exercising, including:

- Excessive fatigue; dizziness
- Palpitations; shortness of breath
- Pain – particularly in the back and pubic areas
- Contractions (*if persistent)
- *Bleeding – seek medical advice

- *Rupture of membranes.

Seek medical advice (*immediately).

### ACOG guidelines (ACOG 1994)

Moderate exercise is defined by the ACOG as brief submaximal maternal exercise up to approximately 70% of maternal aerobic power (ACOG 1994):

- Women should avoid exercise in the supine position after the first trimester. Such a position is associated with decreased cardiac output in most pregnant women.
- Pregnant women who exercise in the first trimester should augment heat dissipation by ensuring adequate hydration, appropriate clothing and optimal environmental surroundings during exercise.
- Many of the physiological and morphological changes of pregnancy persist 4–6 weeks postpartum. Thus pre-pregnancy exercise routines should be resumed gradually based on a woman's physical capability.

### Additional comment from the researcher

The researcher would recommend that current guidelines were adopted during any further research studies in this field of interest. The value of using heart rate or RPE as tools for monitoring exercise intensity has been questioned. Heart rate monitoring should be used only as a guide. Combining heart rate monitoring with some other assessment, such as RPE or the 'talk test', would be more valuable to monitor the level of intensity with individual women during exercise.

# Summary

In the absence of either obstetric or medical complications, pregnant women can continue to exercise and derive related benefits. Women who have achieved cardiovascular fitness before pregnancy should be able to maintain that level of fitness safely throughout pregnancy and the postpartum period (Cheng 1996).

This chapter has provided further information about antenatal and postnatal exercise programmes including the precautions and contraindications. In addition the guidelines for exercise during pregnancy are detailed. This includes the actual guidelines followed in the present study and also the more recent guidelines for the reader's information. The recent guidelines would now be recommended for any reader undertaking research in this field of interest.

# Chapter 4

# Results

This chapter describes the analyses carried out and reports on the results from the randomized controlled study of healthy first-time prospective mothers during and after pregnancy. The control group of participants continued with the existing antenatal preparation for pregnancy, childbirth and the transition to motherhood. In addition, the intervention group participated in a structured antenatal and postnatal exercise programme. The analyses and findings are provided in four separate sections, each reporting on different and related aspects of the study.

The first section presents the findings related to demographic details, baseline information obtained in early pregnancy, and recruitment and retention of participants. The second section details the analyses and findings of the psychological indicators of interest during and after pregnancy. The amount and direction of change in the psychological indicators were of interest during and after pregnancy both between the two groups and within each of the two groups. The third section provides the findings on pregnancy and birth outcomes for both the participants who completed the study and those who dropped out of the study. Finally, the fourth section reports on the aspects related to the physical activity in relation to the frequency, type and correlation with the psychological indicators.

## Analyses

All analyses were carried out using the Minitab Statistics Package. The types of statistical tests carried out depended on the outcome variables being investigated and included repeated measure analyses of variance (ANOVAs), Pearson's product–moment coefficient of correlation analysis, two-sample $t$-tests and chi-squared tests.

Repeated measure ANOVAs were carried out to investigate differences between the groups at the time points of interest during and after pregnancy. Two-sample $t$-tests were undertaken between the two groups with each of the outcome variables in early pregnancy. This allowed baseline comparisons of each of the outcome variables between the two groups before the intervention began.

Two-sample $t$-tests were undertaken to compare mean values of outcome variables measured only once during the study, such as length of gestation, duration of labour, birthweight and episodes of physical activity. Chi-squared tests were undertaken to compare the two groups in relation to demographic details: length of gestation, duration of labour, mode of delivery, Apgar scores, birthweight, postnatal emotional well-being, activity levels and participants who dropped out of the study. Correlation analyses were undertaken after pregnancy using Pearson's product–moment coefficient of correlation, to determine whether there was a relationship between the frequency of total activity and the responses of the three psychological indicators.

More detailed information about individual statistical tests is provided in the relevant sections. Analyses were carried out following advice from a statistician in the Statistics Department, University of Glasgow.

## Participants

Participants were first-time prospective mothers who attended the antenatal clinic at Ayrshire Central Hospital, Irvine for their first antenatal appointment in early pregnancy. All participants recruited to the study were healthy women with no history of medical conditions or previous miscarriage, and who had had an uneventful and healthy pregnancy at the time of recruitment. Findings reported in this section include information about the participants in relation to the recruitment for the study, age, marital status, employment status and levels of activity reported in early pregnancy. This information was obtained from the participants at the time of recruitment to the study.

The control group continued with the existing antenatal education programme during and after pregnancy whereas the intervention group had, in addition, a structured antenatal and postnatal exercise programme. The number and percentages of participants in each group, who were recruited to the study, dropped out of the study and completed the study, are presented in Table 4.1.

A total of 75 participants were recruited to the control group, of whom 48 (64%) completed the study. A total of 82 participants were recruited to the intervention group, of whom 50 (61%) completed the study.

**Table 4.1** Number of participants in each group who were recruited, dropped out or completed the study

| Group | Number recruited | Number (%) who dropped out: | | Number (%) completed |
|---|---|---|---|---|
| | | Immediately | During | |
| Control | 75 | 22 (29) | 5 (7) | 48 (64) |
| Exercise | 82 | 27 (33) | 5 (6) | 50 (61) |
| Overall | 157 | 49 (32) | 10 (6) | 98 (62) |

The drop-out rate of participants from each group was the highest level following recruitment after consent was obtained and before any data were collected, i.e. 22 (29%) from the control group and 27 (33%) from the intervention group. Thereafter, the drop-out rate from each group was minimal during the remainder of the study, i.e. control group 5 (7%) and intervention group 5 (6%).

The age range, mean age, and the number and percentage of participants in each age group are presented in Table 4.2. The age range and mean age of participants in the two groups were comparable, and a chi-squared test indicated that the two groups were not significantly different in relation to the number of participants within each age group. The average age was 28 years for the participants in the control group and 27 years for those in the intervention group. Most participants in both groups were noted to be between 26 and 35 years of age.

**Table 4.2** Age range and mean age of participants and number in each age group

| Group | Age (years) | | <20 | 21–25 | 26–30 | 31–35 | >35 |
|---|---|---|---|---|---|---|---|
| Control (n = 75) | Range 17–38 | Mean 28 (SD 5) | 5 (7) | 10 (13) | 35 (47) | 20 (26) | 5 (7) |
| Exercise (n = 82) | 17–36 | 26 (SD 7) | 7 (8) | 13 (16) | 34 (42) | 24 (29) | 4 (5) |
| | | | Chi-squared test, $p \geq 0.05$ | | | | |

Percentages are given in parentheses except where standard deviation (SD) is indicated.

The number of participants in both groups in terms of relationship status and employment status are presented in Table 4.3. Of the participants in the control group, 45 (60%) were married and 65 (94%) were in employment. In the intervention group, 50 (61%) of the participants were married and 61 (74%) were in employment. A chi-squared test undertaken indicated that the two groups were not significantly different in terms of relationship status and employment status.

At the time of recruitment in early pregnancy, participants were asked to describe their levels of activity, i.e. inactive, if they did not take any form of physical activity; occasionally active, if activity was not undertaken on any regular basis; regularly active, if they had set episodes of activity a week; and very active, if they exercised more than three times a week. Information was obtained from 53 participants in the control group and 55 participants in the intervention group. The number of participants in each group, within each of the four classifications of activity levels reported in early pregnancy, is presented in Table 4.4.

**Table 4.3** Number of participants in each group in terms of relationship and employment status

| Group | Relationship status | | | Employment status | | |
|---|---|---|---|---|---|---|
| | Married | Partner | Single | Employed | Unemployed | Student |
| Control (n = 75) | 45 (60) | 18 (24) | 12 (16) | 65 (94) | 10 (6) | 0 (0) |
| Exercise (n = 82) | 50 (61) | 25 (30) | 7 (9) | 61 (74) | 18 (22) | 3 (4) |
| | Chi-squared test, $p \geq 0.05$ | | | Chi-squared test, $p \geq 0.05$ | | |

Percentages are given in parentheses.

**Table 4.4** Classification of activity levels at time of recruitment for the number of participants in each group

| Group | Classification of activity levels at time of recruitment (early pregnancy) | | | |
|---|---|---|---|---|
| | Inactive | Occasionally active | Regularly active | Very active |
| Control (n = 53) | 14 (26) | 28 (53) | 8 (15) | 3 (6) |
| Exercise (n = 55) | 9 (16) | 33 (60) | 7 (13) | 6 (11) |
| | Chi-squared test, $p \geq 0.05$ | | | |

Percentages are given in parentheses.

Inactivity was reported by 14 (26%) of the participants in the control group and 9 (16%) of the participants in the intervention group. Most of the participants in each group reported being active only on occasion, i.e. 28 (53%) in the control group and 33 (60%) in the intervention group. A chi-squared test was undertaken, which indicated that both groups were not significantly different in relation to the perceived levels of activity reported in early pregnancy. It was not possible to follow the information about how the participants perceived themselves to be in relation to levels of activity during each stage of the study because of the lack of information provided on the return questionnaires. Participants consistently omitted to provide this information, although it was requested on the questionnaire (see Appendix 10). This was a limitation in the design of the questionnaire because participants assumed that the episodes of activity reported in the activity diary would provide the researcher with this information.

In summary, no differences were found between the participants in the control group and intervention group in relation to age, relationship status, employment status and the perceived levels of activity undertaken in early pregnancy.

The next section reports on the findings of the psychological indicators of well-being that were of interest during each stage of the study.

## Psychological indicators

This section focuses on the findings of the psychological indicators of well-being. On the whole, a similar trend emerged in the findings over the indicators of well-being for the participants in the control group and those in the intervention group. It would be easy to present these findings in some general way to avoid repetition for the reader. However, this could omit minor differences also found within these findings. First, it is proposed to present a general overview of the statistical tests and the initial findings. Thereafter, the findings for each psychological indicator are presented separately to ensure that the reader gains an accurate interpretation of the findings.

The results are reported on the psychological indicators, each measured at the three time points of interest (i.e. early, late and after pregnancy). The information was obtained from two 'self-report' questionnaires to assess psychological well-being, i.e. the psychological well-being questionnaire developed and validated by Moses et al. (1989) and the Maternal Adjustment and Attitude (MAMA) questionnaire by Kumar et al. (1984). The psychological indicators reported include:

- Perceptions of coping assets (positive psychological well-being)
- Perceptions of coping deficits (negative psychological well-being)
- Perceptions of physical well-being
- Perceptions of body image
- Perceptions of somatic symptoms
- Attitudes to marital relationships
- Attitude to sex
- Attitude to pregnancy/baby.

The results are reported on postnatal emotional well-being measured in the postnatal period by the Edinburgh Postnatal Depression Scale, developed by Cox et al. (1987).

## Analysis

Repeated measure ANOVAs were carried out to investigate differences between the *exercise groups* (i.e. two levels – exercise and control) at the *time* points (i.e. three levels – early, late and after pregnancy). The Minitab GLM (General Linear Model) command was used to carry out the repeated measure ANOVAs. The time points of interest were: early pregnancy (12–16 weeks), late pregnancy (36–40 weeks) and after pregnancy (12–16 weeks). Significance level used was $p < 0.05$.

A follow-up multiple-comparison procedure with a simultaneous 95% Confidence Interval (95%CI) was undertaken if a significant *interaction* of time and exercise group was found. The main effects of exercise group or time were of limited interest when there was found to be a significant exercise group/time interaction because the groups were expected to be comparable in early pregnancy. This exercise group/time interaction was of prime importance because the two groups were 'expected' to be similar in early pregnancy and thus a significant interaction would arise as a result of the intervention, where the difference between the two groups would manifest themselves only in late pregnancy and after pregnancy. As a result of this exercise group/time interaction, any overall differences (i.e. averaged over early, late and after pregnancy values) would be of limited interest for the main effect of the exercise group, because they should be similar in early pregnancy. This limited interest was similar for the main effect of time (i.e. averaged across the exercise and control group) because the patterns of the two groups across time were different. Thus, a significant exercise group/time interaction superseded any other (main) effect. The follow-up tests allowed further, more detailed investigation of any differences between the groups for each of the outcome variables measured in the amount of change reported from early (12–16 weeks) to late (36–40 weeks) pregnancy, early (12–16 weeks) to after (12–16 weeks) pregnancy, and late (36–40 weeks) to after (12–16 weeks) pregnancy.

Repeated measure ANOVAs showed a significant interaction ($p < 0.001$) between the two groups and three time points with each of the psychological indicators. Similar interaction was found with each of the psychological indicators over the three time points of interest. This interaction was a key result which indicated that any differences between the two groups in terms of the scores for each of the psychological indicators were not the same at the three time points for the two groups, i.e. early, late and after pregnancy. Table 4.5 presents a summary of the ANOVA results for all the psychological indicators over the three time points. The interaction depicting each separate psychological indicator is presented within the relevant figures presented in each section of these results.

**Table 4.5** Summary of ANOVA results for psychological indicators across all three time points

| Psychological indicator | Exercise group ($p$-value) | Time ($p$-value) | Exercise group time ($p$-value) |
|---|---|---|---|
| **Perceptions of:** | | | |
| Coping assets (positive psychological well-being) | 0.027 | 0.004 | 0.000 |
| Coping deficits (negative psychological well-being) | 0.001 | 0.001 | 0.000 |
| Physical well-being | 0.001 | 0.001 | 0.000 |
| Body image | 0.818 | 0.000 | 0.000 |
| Somatic symptoms | 0.299 | 0.000 | 0.000 |
| **Attitudes to:** | | | |
| Marital relationships | 0.871 | 0.000 | 0.000 |
| Sex | 0.138 | 0.000 | 0.000 |
| Pregnancy/baby | 0.054 | 0.000 | 0.000 |

## Perceptions of coping assets

Perceptions of coping assets (positive psychological well-being) predominantly contained positive statements and feelings of 'self'. An increase in scores indicated a more positive perception in the ability to cope. In contrast, more negative perceptions were denoted by a decrease in scores, i.e. a reduction in the perceived ability to cope.

Repeated measure ANOVAs showed a significant interaction ($p < 0.001$) between the two groups and three time points. The interaction is depicted in Figure 4.1 and was a key result. This indicated that any differences between the two groups in terms of the scores for

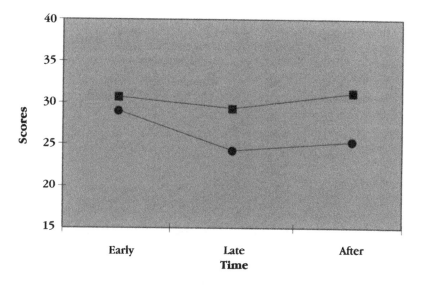

**Figure 4.1** Mean scores for perceptions of coping assets (positive psychological well-being). ● Control group; ■ Exercise group.

perceptions of coping assets (positive psychological well-being) were not the same at the three time points for the two groups, i.e. early, late and after pregnancy.

Mean scores and standard deviations for both groups at each time point are shown in Table 4.6 along with significance of the differences established by between-group follow-up tests. The follow-up tests indicated that there was no difference between the two groups in early pregnancy, but significant differences were noted in both late pregnancy and after pregnancy.

Follow-up analysis involving two-sample $t$-tests and 95%CI were then calculated on the changes for each group from early to late pregnancy, late to after pregnancy and from early to after pregnancy. These are shown in Table 4.7.

**Table 4.6** Mean (standard deviation or SD) scores for perceptions of coping assets in early, late and after pregnancy with between-group follow-up tests and $p$-values

| Group | Early pregnancy | Late pregnancy | After pregnancy |
| --- | --- | --- | --- |
| Control | 29.8 (8.9) | 24.1 (9.2) | 25.6 (10.2) |
| Exercise | 30.4 (8.9) | 28.9 (9.4) | 31.1 (9.0) |
| $p$-value | 0.17 | 0.02 | 0.01 |

**Table 4.7** Follow-up multiple-comparison tests for perceptions of coping assets

| Changes from: | | Early pregnancy | | Late pregnancy |
|---|---|---|---|---|
| Group | | Late minus early | After minus early | After minus late |
| Control | Mean (SD) | −6.8 (9.6) | −4.8 (10.5) | +1.6 (9.8) |
| | 95%CI | −9.9, −3.7 | −8.2, −1.3 | −1.7, 4.8 |
| Exercise | Mean (SD) | +0.2 (7.7) | +2.1 (7.7) | +1.6 (7.4) |
| | 95%CI | −2.1, 2.6 | −0.2, 4.4 | −0.6, 3.8 |
| Exercise minus control | Difference | 7.0 | 6.9 | 0 |
| | 95%CI | 3.2, 10.9 | 2.7, 10.9 | −3.8, 3.9 |
| | $p$-value | < 0.001 | < 0.001 | > 0.05 |

On the perception of coping assets scale, there was a significant difference found between the two groups in the amount of change from early to late pregnancy; the control group showed a significant decrease whereas the exercise group showed no significant change during the same period.

A significant difference was found between the groups in the amount of change from early to after pregnancy; the control group again showed a significant decrease in scores on average during this period, whereas there was no evidence of change within the exercise group during and after pregnancy.

No significant difference was found between the groups in the amount of change from late to after pregnancy. There was found to be no significant change, on average, within either of the groups during this period.

From the findings, it can be concluded that the participants in the intervention group showed, on average, maintenance in the perceptions of coping assets from early to after pregnancy. This was in contrast to the participants in the control group, who showed a significant decrease in the perceptions of coping assets during the same period.

## Perceptions of coping deficits

Perceptions of coping deficits (negative psychological well-being) consisted predominantly of negative feelings and poor competence. An increase in the coping deficits score indicated a negative response in perceptions of deficits in the ability to cope. In contrast, if the score decreased, this indicated a reduction in perceptions of deficits in coping, which signified a more positive response.

Repeated measure ANOVAs showed a significant interaction ($p < 0.001$) between the two groups and three time points. The interaction is depicted in Figure 4.2 and was a key result. This indicated that any differences between the two groups in terms of the scores for perceptions of coping deficits (negative psychological well-being) were not the same at the three time points for the two groups, i.e. early, late and after pregnancy.

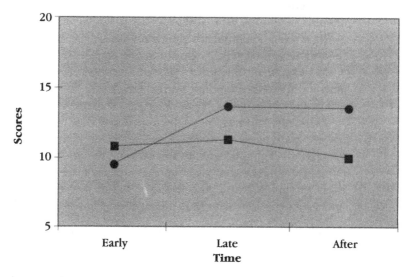

**Figure 4.2** Mean scores of perceptions of coping deficits (negative psychological well-being). ● Control group; ■ Exercise group.

Mean scores and standard deviations for both groups at each time point are shown in Table 4.8, along with the level of significance of the differences established by between-group follow-up tests. The follow-up tests indicated that there was no difference between the two groups in both early pregnancy and late pregnancy, but there was a significant difference noted after pregnancy.

Follow-up analysis involving two-sample $t$-tests and 95%CI were then calculated on the changes for each group from early to late

**Table 4.8** Mean (SD) scores for perceptions of coping deficits in early, late and after pregnancy with between-group follow-up tests and $p$-values

| Group | Early pregnancy | Late pregnancy | After pregnancy |
|---|---|---|---|
| Control | 9.7 (3.7) | 14.4 (6.9) | 14.0 (6.9) |
| Exercise | 10.8 (5.2) | 11.7 (6.5) | 10.2 (6.8) |
| $p$-value | 0.24 | 0.17 | 0.01 |

pregnancy, late to after pregnancy and early to after pregnancy. These are shown in Table 4.9.

On the perceptions of coping deficits scale, there was a significant difference found between the two groups in the amount of change from early to late pregnancy; the control group showed a significant increase whereas the intervention group showed no significant change during the same period.

A significant difference was found between the two groups in the amount of change from early to after pregnancy; the control group again showed a significant increase whereas the intervention group showed no significant change during the same period.

No significant difference was found between the two groups in the amount of change from late to after pregnancy. No significant change was found within either of the two groups during this period.

From the findings, it can be concluded that participants in the intervention group experienced no significant change, on average, in perceptions of coping deficits from early to after pregnancy. In contrast, participants in the control group experienced a significant increase in their perceptions of coping deficits, which was more negative and indicated perceived deficits in coping during and after pregnancy.

**Table 4.9** Follow-up multiple-comparison tests for perceptions of coping deficits

| Changes from: | | Early pregnancy | | Late pregnancy |
|---|---|---|---|---|
| Group | | Late minus early | After minus early | After minus late |
| 1. Control | Mean (SD) | +5.2  (6.5) | +4.4  (7.9) | −0.8  (8.8) |
| | 95%CI | 3.1,  7.3 | 1.8,  7.0 | −3.7,  2.0 |
| 2. Exercise | Mean (SD) | +0.3  (5.1) | −1.1  (6.4) | −1.3  (5.6) |
| | 95%CI | −1.2,  1.8 | −3.0,  0.8 | −2.9,  0.3 |
| Exercise | Difference | −4.9 | −5.5 | −0.5 |
| minus | 95%CI | −7.5, −2.4 | −8.7,−2.3 | −3.7,  2.7 |
| Control | | | | |
| | p-value | < 0.001 | < 0.001 | > 0.05 |

## Perceptions of physical well-being

Perceptions of physical well-being predominantly contained statements about physical well-being, e.g. feelings of being healthy, strong, supple, etc. An increase in scores indicated a more positive perception in physical well-being, whereas negative perceptions of physical well-being were denoted by a decrease in scores.

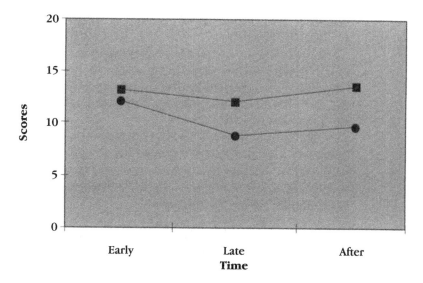

**Figure 4.3** Mean scores of perceptions of physical well-being. ● Control group; ■ Exercise group.

Repeated measure ANOVAs showed a significant interaction ($p < 0.001$) between the two groups and three time points. The interaction is depicted in Figure 4.3 and was a key result. This indicated that any differences between the two groups in terms of the scores for perceptions of coping assets were not the same at the three time points for the two groups, i.e. early, late and after pregnancy.

Mean scores and standard deviations for both groups at each time point are shown in Table 4.10, along with the level of significance of the differences established by between-group follow-up tests. The follow-up tests indicated that there was no difference between the two groups in early pregnancy, but significant differences were noted in both late pregnancy and after pregnancy.

Follow-up analysis involving two-sample $t$-tests and 95%CI values were then calculated on the changes for each group from early to late

**Table 4.10** Mean (SD) scores for perceptions of physical well-being in early, late and after pregnancy with between-group follow-up tests and $p$-values

| Group | Early pregnancy | Late pregnancy | After pregnancy |
|---|---|---|---|
| Control | 11.5 (3.4) | 8.3 (4.4) | 9.6 (4.9) |
| Exercise | 12.8 (3.4) | 11.7 (4.8) | 12.6 (4.1) |
| $p$-value | 0.12 | 0.00 | 0.00 |

pregnancy, late to after pregnancy and early to after pregnancy. These are shown in Table 4.11.

On the perception of physical well-being scale, there was a significant difference found between the two groups in the amount of change from early to late pregnancy; the control group showed a significant decrease whereas the intervention group showed no significant change during the same period.

A significant difference was found between the amount of change from early to after pregnancy between the groups; the control group again showed a significant decrease in scores on average during this period, although there was no evidence of change within the intervention group during and after pregnancy.

No significant difference was found between the groups in the amount of change from late to after pregnancy. No significant change, on average, was found within either of the two groups during this period.

From the findings, it can be concluded that the participants in the intervention group experienced, on average, maintenance in the perceptions of physical well-being from early to after pregnancy. This was in contrast to the participants in the control group, who experienced a significant decrease in the perceptions of physical well-being during the same period.

**Table 4.11** Follow-up multiple-comparison tests for perceptions of physical well-being

| Changes from: | | Early pregnancy | | Late pregnancy |
|---|---|---|---|---|
| Group | | Late minus early | After minus early | After minus late |
| Control | Mean (SD) | −3.8 (4.9) | −2.9 (5.6) | +0.9 (4.6) |
| | 95% CI | −5.4, −2.2 | −4.7, −1.1 | −0.6, 2.4 |
| Exercise | Mean (SD) | −0.1 (4.7) | +0.6 (4.9) | +0.9 (4.8) |
| | 95% CI | −1.5, 1.3 | −0.8, 2.1 | −0.6, 2.3 |
| Exercise minus Control | Difference | 3.7 | 2.3 | 0 |
| | 95% CI | 1.6, 5.8 | 1.2, 3.5 | −2.0, 2.0 |
| | $p$-value | < 0.001 | < 0.01 | > 0.05 |

**Perceptions of body image**

Perceptions of body image predominantly consisted of statements about perceived attractiveness, body shape, and to what extent women were pleased or disappointed in the shape of their body during and after pregnancy. An increase in scores indicated more positive perceptions

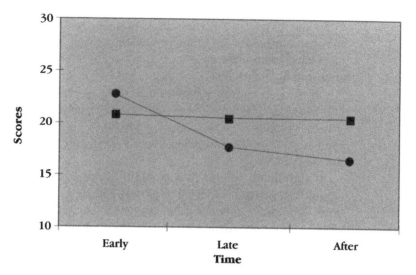

**Figure 4.4** Mean scores for perceptions of body image. ● Control group; ■ Exercise group.

in body image whereas more negative perceptions in body image were denoted by a decrease in scores.

Repeated measure ANOVAs showed a significant interaction ($p < 0.001$) between the two groups and three time points. The interaction is depicted in Figure 4.4 and was a key result. This indicated that any differences between the two groups in terms of the scores for perceptions of body image were not the same at the three time points for the two groups, i.e. early, late and after pregnancy.

Mean scores and standard deviations for both groups at each time point are shown in Table 4.12, along with significance of the differences established by between-group follow-up tests. The follow-up tests indicated that there were significant differences between the two groups in early pregnancy, late pregnancy and after pregnancy. In early pregnancy, the control group had significantly higher scores and more positive scores than the intervention group. In late pregnancy and after pregnancy, the intervention group had significantly higher and more positive scores than the control group.

**Table 4.12** Mean (SD) scores for perceptions of body image in early, late and after pregnancy with between-group follow-up tests and $p$-values

| Group | Early pregnancy | Late pregnancy | After pregnancy |
|---|---|---|---|
| Control | 22.9 (3.3) | 17.6 (5.2) | 16.1 (4.4) |
| Exercise | 20.7 (5.2) | 20.2 (5.1) | 20.0 (5.7) |
| $p$-value | 0.03 | 0.01 | 0.00 |

Follow-up analysis involving two-sample $t$-tests and 95%CI were then calculated on the changes for each group from early to late pregnancy, late to after pregnancy and early to after pregnancy. These are shown in Table 4.13.

On the perception of body image scale, there was a significant difference found between the two groups in the amount of change from early to late pregnancy; the control group showed a significant decrease whereas the intervention group showed no significant change during the same period.

A significant difference was found between the groups in the amount of change from early to after pregnancy; the control group again showed a significant decrease in scores on average during this period. In contrast, there was no evidence of change within the intervention group during and after pregnancy.

No significant difference was found between the groups in the amount of change from late to after pregnancy. There was noted to be a significant decrease in the amount of change within the control group during this same period.

From the findings, it can be concluded that the participants in the intervention group showed, on average, maintenance in the perceptions of body image from early to after pregnancy. This was in contrast to the participants in the control group, who showed a significant decrease in the perceptions of body image during the same period.

**Table 4.13** Follow-up multiple-comparison tests for perceptions of body image

| Changes from: | | Early pregnancy | | Late pregnancy |
|---|---|---|---|---|
| Group | | Late minus early | After minus early | After minus late |
| Control | Mean (SD) | −6.2 (7.4) | −8.5 (8.6) | −2.2 (5.3) |
| | 95%CI | −8.8, −3.6 | −11.5, −5.6 | −4.0, −0.4 |
| Exercise | Mean (SD) | −0.5 (4.8) | −0.5 (5.6) | −0.4 (5.8) |
| | 95%CI | −1.9, 1.0 | −2.2, 1.1 | −2.2, 1.3 |
| Exercise minus Control | Difference | 5.7 | 8.0 | 1.8 |
| | 95%CI | 2.8, 8.6 | 4.7, 11.4 | −0.7, 4.2 |
| | $p$-value | < 0.001 | < 0.001 | > 0.05 |

## Perceptions of somatic symptoms

Somatic symptoms experienced during pregnancy are those symptoms that affect the body in terms of health and well-being. These include feelings of nausea and vomiting, constipation, swollen ankles, fainting and light-headedness, fatigue and tiredness.

Perceptions of somatic symptoms predominantly contained statements about the extent to which somatic symptoms were experienced. An increase in scores indicated a more positive perception in the extent to which somatic symptoms were experienced whereas more negative perceptions were denoted by a decrease in scores, i.e. somatic symptoms were experienced to a greater extent.

Repeated measure ANOVAs showed a significant interaction ($p < 0.001$) between the two groups and three time points. The interaction is depicted in Figure 4.5 and was a key result. This indicated that any differences between the two groups in terms of the scores for perceptions of somatic symptoms were not the same at the three time points for the two groups, i.e. early, late and after pregnancy.

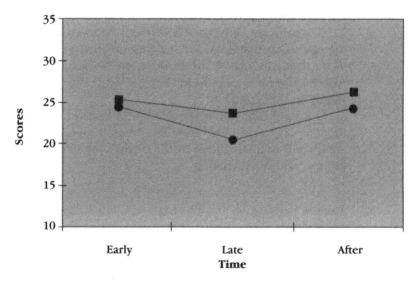

**Figure 4.5** Mean scores for perceptions of somatic symptoms. ● Control group; ■ Exercise group.

Mean scores and standard deviations for both groups at each time point are shown in Table 4.14, along with significance of the differences established by between-group follow-up tests. The follow-up tests indicated that there was no difference between the two groups in early pregnancy, although significant differences were noted both in late pregnancy and after pregnancy.

Follow-up analysis involving two-sample $t$-tests and 95%CI were then calculated on the changes for each group from early to late

**Table 4.14** Mean (SD) scores for perceptions of somatic symptoms in early, late and after pregnancy with between-group follow-up tests and p-values

| Group | Early pregnancy | Late pregnancy | After pregnancy |
|---|---|---|---|
| Control | 24.7 (4.6) | 20.1 (5.5) | 24.5 (4.6) |
| Exercise | 25.6 (4.6) | 23.9 (4.2) | 27.0 (4.1) |
| p-value | 0.25 | 0.01 | 0.01 |

pregnancy, late to after pregnancy and early to after pregnancy. These are shown in Table 4.15.

On the perception of somatic symptoms scale, there was a significant difference found between the two groups in the amount of change from early to late pregnancy; the control group showed a significant decrease whereas the intervention group showed no significant change during the same period.

A significant difference was found between the groups in the amount of change from early to after pregnancy; the control group again showed a significant decrease, on average, during this period whereas there was a significant increase within the intervention group during and after pregnancy.

No significant difference was found between the groups in the amount of change noted from late to after pregnancy. There was a significant increase found in the change, on average, within both groups during this period.

**Table 4.15** Follow-up multiple-comparison tests for perceptions of somatic symptoms

| Changes from: | | Early pregnancy | | Late pregnancy |
|---|---|---|---|---|
| Group | | Late minus early | After minus early | After minus late |
| Control | Mean (SD) | −5.3 (7.1) | −0.6 (7.2) | +4.7 (5.4) |
| | 95%CI | −7.7, −3.0 | −2.9, 1.7 | 2.8, 6.5 |
| Exercise | Mean (SD) | −0.1 (5.7) | +3.4 (5.4) | +3.6 (4.7) |
| | 95%CI | −1.8, 1.7 | 1.8, 5.0 | 2.1, 5.0 |
| Exercise minus Control | Difference | 5.2 | 2.8 | 1.1 |
| | 95%CI | 2.4, 8.2 | 1.2, 6.8 | −3.4, 1.2 |
| | p-value | < 0.001 | < 0.01 | > 0.05 |

From the findings, it can be concluded that the participants in the intervention group showed, on average, maintenance in the perceptions of somatic symptoms from early to after pregnancy, which was in contrast to the participants in the control group, who showed a significant increase in the perceptions of somatic symptoms during the same period.

### Attitudes to marital relationships

Higher scores indicated a positive attitude to marital relationships. Therefore, an increase in scores indicated a more positive attitude to marital relationships whereas more negative attitudes to marital relationships were denoted by a decrease in scores.

Repeated measure ANOVAs showed a significant interaction ($p < 0.001$) between the two groups and three time points. The interaction is depicted in Figure 4.6 and was a key result. This indicated that any differences between the two groups in terms of the scores for attitudes to marital relationships were not the same at the three time points for the two groups, i.e. early, late and after pregnancy.

Mean scores and standard deviations for both groups at each time point are shown in Table 4.16, along with significance of the differences established by between-group follow-up tests. The follow-up tests indicated that there was no difference between the two groups in early pregnancy and late pregnancy, but a significant difference was noted after pregnancy.

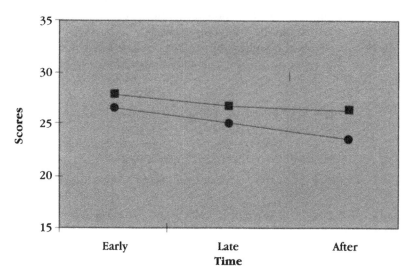

**Figure 4.6** Mean scores of attitude to marital relationships. ● Control group; ■ Exercise group.

**Table 4.16** Mean (SD) scores for attitudes to marital relationships in early, late and after pregnancy with between-group follow-up tests and p-values

| Group | Early pregnancy | Late pregnancy | After pregnancy |
|---|---|---|---|
| Control | 27.1 (5.8) | 25.1 (5.4) | 22.8 (5.8) |
| Exercise | 28.3 (5.9) | 27.2 (5.4) | 26.1 (6.2) |
| p-value | 0.15 | 0.17 | 0.01 |

Follow-up analysis involving two-sample t-tests and 95%CI were then calculated on the changes for each group from early to late pregnancy, late to after pregnancy and early to after pregnancy. These are shown in Table 4.17.

On the attitudes to marital relationships scale, there was no significant difference found between the two groups in the amount of change from early to late pregnancy. The control group showed a significant decrease in attitudes to marital relationships, whereas the intervention group showed no significant change during the same period.

A significant difference was found between the two groups in the amount of change from early to after pregnancy; both groups showed a significant decrease in scores on average during and after pregnancy.

No significant difference was noted between the groups in the amount of change found from late to after pregnancy. The control group continued to show a significant decrease whereas no difference was found in the intervention group.

From the findings, it can be concluded that there was a significant difference in the amount of average change in attitudes to marital

**Table 4.17** Follow-up multiple-comparison tests for attitudes to marital relationships

| Changes from: | | Early pregnancy | | Late pregnancy |
|---|---|---|---|---|
| Group | | Late minus early | After minus early | After minus late |
| Control | Mean (SD) | −2.1 (5.8) | −1.8 (4.9) | −4.0 (6.5) |
| | 95%CI | −4.0, −0.2 | −7.5, −4.4 | −6.2, −1.9 |
| Exercise | Mean (SD) | −1.2 (4.1) | −3.9 (4.9) | −1.0 (4.8) |
| | 95%CI | −2.4, 0.1 | −3.4, −0.3 | −2.4, 0.5 |
| Exercise | Difference | 0.9 | 4.1 | 3.0 |
| minus | 95%CI | −1.3, 3.2 | 2.0, 6.2 | 0.5, 5.6 |
| Control | | | | |
| | p-value | > 0.05 | < 0.001 | < 0.05 |

relationships during and after pregnancy, with both groups demon-strating a significant decrease in their attitude to marital relationships throughout this period. Although both groups followed a similar pattern of decrease in their attitudes to marital relationships, the inter-vention group tended to decrease to a lesser extent than the control group and maintained more positive attitudes to marital relationships both during and after pregnancy.

### Attitudes to sex

Higher scores indicated a positive attitude towards sex. Therefore, an increase in scores indicated a more positive attitude to sex whereas more negative attitudes to sex were denoted by a subsequent decrease in scores.

Repeated measure ANOVAs showed a significant interaction ($p < 0.001$) between the two groups and three time points. The interac-tion is depicted in Figure 4.7 and was a key result. This indicated that any differences between the two groups in terms of the scores for attitudes to sex were not the same at the three time points for the two groups, i.e. early, late and after pregnancy.

The mean scores and standard deviations for both groups at each time point are shown in Table 4.18, along with significance of the differences established by between-group follow-up tests. The follow-up tests indicated that there was no difference between the two groups

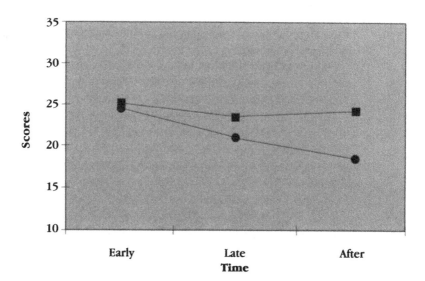

**Figure 4.7** Mean scores of attitudes to sex. ● Control group; ■ Exercise group.

**Table 4.18** Mean (SD) scores for attitudes to sex in early, late and after pregnancy with between-group follow-up tests and p-values

| Group | Early pregnancy | Late pregnancy | After pregnancy |
|---|---|---|---|
| Control | 24.5 (5.8) | 21.0 (6.9) | 18.2 (7.9) |
| Exercise | 25.2 (5.7) | 23.5 (6.0) | 23.7 (5.4) |
| p-value | 0.35 | 0.29 | 0.01 |

**Table 4.19** Follow-up multiple-comparison tests for attitudes to sex

| Changes from: | | Early pregnancy | | Late pregnancy |
|---|---|---|---|---|
| Group | | Late minus early | After minus early | After minus late |
| Control | Mean (SD) | −4.7 (6.9) | −7.9 (9.4) | −3.0 (6.7) |
| | 95%CI | −7.0, −2.3 | −11.1, −4.6 | −5.4, −0.7 |
| Exercise | Mean (SD) | −0.6 (4.2) | −0.3 (5.4) | −0.02 (6.2) |
| | 95%CI | −2.0, 0.7 | −1.9, 1.4 | −1.9, 1.8 |
| Exercise minus Control | Difference | 4.1 | 7.6 | 2.98 |
| | 95%CI | 1.4, 6.7 | 4.0, 11.2 | 0.1, 6.0 |
| | p-value | < 0.01 | < 0.001 | ≥ 0.05 |

in early pregnancy or late pregnancy, but a significant difference was noted after pregnancy.

Follow-up two-sample t-tests and 95%CI were then calculated on the changes for each group from early to late pregnancy, late to after pregnancy and early to after pregnancy. These are shown in Table 4.19.

On the attitudes to sex scale, there was a significant difference found between the two groups in the amount of change from early to late pregnancy; the control group showed a significant decrease whereas the intervention group showed no significant change during the same period.

A significant difference was noted between the groups in the amount of change from early to after pregnancy; the control group again showed a significant decrease in scores on average during this period, whereas there was no significant change noted within the intervention group during and after pregnancy.

No difference was found between the groups in the amount of change from late to after pregnancy. The control group continued to

experience significant decrease in attitudes to sex whereas no significant change was noted within the intervention group over this period.

From the findings, it can be concluded that the participants in the
intervention group experienced, on average, a maintenance in the
attitudes to sex from early to after pregnancy, which was in contrast to
the participants in the control group, who experienced a significant
decrease in the attitudes to sex during the same period.

### Attitudes to pregnancy/baby

Positive attitudes to pregnancy/baby are indicated by higher scores.
Therefore, an increase in scores during pregnancy indicated a more
positive attitude to pregnancy, whereas negative attitudes were denoted
by a decrease in scores, i.e. more negative attitudes to pregnancy. This
was similar for attitudes to the baby in the period after pregnancy.

Repeated measure ANOVAs showed a significant interaction
($p < 0.001$) between the two groups and three time points. The interaction is depicted in Figure 4.8 and was a key result. This indicated that
any differences between the two groups in terms of the scores for
attitudes to pregnancy/baby were not the same at the three time points
for the two groups, i.e. early, late and after pregnancy.

Mean scores and standard deviations for both groups at each time
point are shown in Table 4.20, along with significance of the differences established by between-group follow-up tests. The follow-up tests

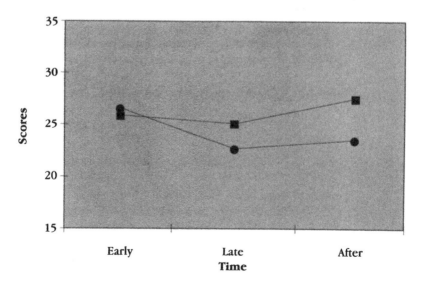

**Figure 4.8** Mean scores for attitude to pregnancy/baby. ● Control group;
■ Exercise group.

**Table 4.20** Mean (SD) scores for attitudes to pregnancy/baby in early, late and after pregnancy with between-group follow-up tests and p-values

| Group | Early pregnancy | Late pregnancy | After pregnancy |
|---|---|---|---|
| Control | 26.6 (3.9) | 22.0 (5.2) | 24.7 (5.1) |
| Exercise | 26.0 (8.9) | 25.2 (9.4) | 28.6 (3.8) |
| p-value | 0.38 | 0.01 | 0.00 |

indicated that there was no difference between the two groups in early pregnancy, although significant differences were noted both in late pregnancy and after pregnancy.

Follow-up analysis involving two-sample t-tests and 95%CI were then calculated on the changes for each group from early to late pregnancy, late to after pregnancy and early to after pregnancy. These are shown in Table 4.21.

On the attitudes to pregnancy/baby scale, a significant difference was found between the two groups in the amount of change from early to late pregnancy; the control group showed a significant decrease whereas the intervention group showed no significant change during the same period.

A significant difference was found between the two groups in the amount of change from early to after pregnancy; the control group again showed a significant decrease in scores on average during this period, whereas there was no evidence of change within the intervention group during and after pregnancy.

No significant difference was noted between the groups in the amount of change found from late to after pregnancy. A significant

**Table 4.21** Follow-up multiple-comparison tests for attitudes to pregnancy/baby

| Changes from: | | Early pregnancy | | Late pregnancy |
|---|---|---|---|---|
| Group | | Late minus early | After minus early | After minus late |
| Control | Mean (SD) | −5.1 (5.6) | −2.2 (6.7) | +2.7 (5.3) |
| | 95%CI | −6.9, −3.3 | −4.4, −0.03 | 0.9, 4.4 |
| Exercise | Mean (SD) | −0.4 (4.6) | +3.3 (4.7) | +3.7 (4.2) |
| | 95%CI | −1.8, 1.0 | −1.9, 4.7 | 2.5, 5.0 |
| Exercise | Difference | 4.7 | 5.5 | 1.0 |
| minus | 95%CI | 2.4, 6.9 | 2.9, 8.1 | −1.1, 3.18 |
| control | | | | |
| | p-value | < 0.001 | < 0.001 | > 0.05 |

positive change, on average, was found within the two groups during this period.

From the findings, it can be concluded that the participants in the intervention group experienced, on average, a maintenance in attitudes to pregnancy/baby from early to after pregnancy, which was in contrast to the participants in the control group, who experienced a significant negative change in attitude to pregnancy during pregnancy with positive significant change in attitudes to the baby after pregnancy.

## Postnatal emotional well-being/depression

Postnatal emotional well-being/depression measured by the Edinburgh Postnatal Depression Scale (EPDS) has a possible range of scores between 0 and 30 points. Lower scores indicate positive emotional well-being with higher scores being more negative and indicating a decrease in emotional well-being states. The measurement tool (EPDS) is a screening tool designed to indicate a tendency towards depressive states with increasing levels of symptoms with scores >12 points (Cox et al. 1987).

From the results obtained, 79 participants obtained scores below 8 points and the remaining 5 participants scored between 8 and 11 points. These scores were divided into three categories (< 4 points, between 5 and 8 points, and > 8 points). The numbers of participants who responded within each of the three categories of scores are presented in Table 4.22. In both groups, a reduced number of participants responded to this particular outcome variable, i.e. 77% ($n = 37$) of the participants in the control group and 94% ($n = 47$) in the intervention group.

The range of scores obtained from participants was between 0 and 11 points for the control group and between 0 and 9 points for the intervention group. Mean score for the control group was 6.4 (SD 1.3) and 4.8 (SD 1.7) for the intervention group. Both groups of participants responded with scores below 11 points, which indicated positive

**Table 4.22** Postnatal emotional well-being/depression scores

| Group | <4 points | 5–8 points | >8 points |
|---|---|---|---|
| Control ($n = 37$)[a] | 7 (19) | 26 (70) | 4 (11) |
| Exercise ($n = 47$)[a] | 16 (34) | 30 (64) | 1 (2) |
| | Chi-squared test, $p \geq 0.05$ | | |

[a]Percentages are given in parentheses.

emotional well-being. These findings suggested that there was no evidence of a tendency towards depressive symptoms because all scores were below 12 points. Most participants in both groups obtained scores between 5 and 8 points, i.e. 70% ($n = 26$) and 64% ($n = 30$) for the control group and intervention group, respectively. Scores below 4 points were obtained from 19% ($n = 7$) of participants in the control group and 34% ($n = 16$) in the intervention group. Only 11% ($n = 4$) of the participants in the control group and 2% ($n = 1$) in the intervention group scored over 8 points.

Findings from a chi-squared test indicated that there was no significant difference between the two groups, although there was a tendency for participants in the intervention group to have lower and more positive scores when compared with those in the control group. These findings indicated that both the groups demonstrated positive responses to postnatal emotional well-being with no evidence of any tendency towards depressive states.

In summary, this section reported the findings of the psychological indicators of well-being. A similar trend in the findings was observed in the psychological indicators studied during and after pregnancy. Psychological indicators of interest included perceptions of positive and negative psychological well-being, physical well-being, body image, somatic symptoms experienced, and attitudes to marital relationships, sex and to both pregnancy and the baby. The findings suggest that participants in regular physical activity during and after pregnancy tended to have no significant changes in levels of psychological well-being both during and after pregnancy. This was in contrast to the participants in the control group who had a significant deterioration in psychological well-being during the same period of time. Participants in both groups experienced positive emotional psychological well-being with no tendency towards expressing depressive feelings.

The next section presents the findings in relation to pregnancy and birth outcomes, for both the participants who completed the study and, where possible, for those who dropped out of the study. This includes the length of gestation, duration of labour, type of delivery, Apgar scores of the baby, birthweight, and any maternal or neonatal complications experienced.

## Pregnancy/birth outcomes

Pregnancy outcomes of interest included the length of gestation, duration of labour, mode of delivery and any maternal complications experienced. Birth outcomes of interest included the Apgar score of the baby at 1 and 5 minutes after birth, birthweight and any neonatal complications arising. This information was obtained from

**Table 4.23** Length of gestation (weeks)

| Group | <37 weeks | 38–40 weeks | >40 weeks |
|---|---|---|---|
| Control (n = 37)[a] | 3 (8) | 23 (62) | 11 (30) |
| Exercise (n = 50)[a] | 4 (8) | 30 (60) | 16 (32) |
| | Chi–squared test, $p \geq 0.05$ | | |

[a]Percentages are given in parentheses.

the questionnaire completed by the participants in the postnatal period or directly from the obstetric case notes when this was necessary. In relation to pregnancy and birth outcome, the amount of information obtained varied for both groups. This ranged from 77% (n = 37) to 100% (n = 48) for the control group and from 90% (n = 45) to 100% (n = 50) for the intervention group. This particular information was either not being provided, or available or accessible to the researcher.

**Length of gestation**

The period of gestation indicates the length or the gestational age of pregnancy, with a normal pregnancy being 40 weeks in duration. Preterm delivery occurs before the completion of week 37 of the pregnancy (Sweet and Tiran 1997).

The number of participants who delivered before 37 weeks, between 38 and 40 weeks and after 40 weeks' gestation is presented in Table 4.23. The range of gestation was between 33 and 42 weeks for participants in both the control and intervention groups. Mean length of gestation was 39.8 (SD 1.6) weeks and 40.1 (1.9) weeks for the control group and intervention group respectively.

Most of the participants in both groups delivered between 38 and 40 weeks' gestation, i.e. 62% (n = 23) for the control group and 60% (n = 30) for the intervention group. Pre-term deliveries were experienced by 8% of participants in both groups, i.e. before completion of week 37 of pregnancy. Findings from a chi-squared test indicated that there was

**Table 4.24** Duration of labour (hours)

| Group | <4 hours | 5–8 hours | >8 hours |
|---|---|---|---|
| Control (n = 37)[a] | 10 (27) | 16 (43) | 11 (30) |
| Exercise (n = 50)[a] | 18 (36) | 24 (48) | 8 (16) |
| | Chi-squared test, $p \geq 0.05$ | | |

[a]Percentages are given in parentheses.

**Table 4.25** Mode of delivery

| Group | n | Normal (SVD) | Instrumental | Surgical |
|---|---|---|---|---|
| Control | 48 | 32 (67) | 12 (25) | 4 (8) |
| Exercise | 50 | 37 (74) | 11 (22) | 2 (4) |
| | | Chi-squared test, $p \geq 0.05$ | | |

Percentages are given in parentheses.

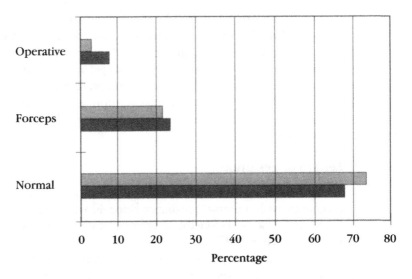

**Figure 4.9** Bar chart of mode of delivery. ☐ Exercise group; ■ Control group.

no significant difference between the two groups in relation to the length of gestation at delivery.

### Duration of labour

The number of participants and duration of labour experienced, i.e. < 4 hours, between 5 and 8 hours, and > 8 hours, is presented in Table 4.24. The range in duration of labour was between 1 and 14 hours for participants in both the control and intervention groups. Average duration of labour was 8.4 (SD 4.7) hours for participants in the control group and 7.6 (3.2) hours for the participants in the intervention group. Most participants in both groups experienced labour of between 5 and 8 hours in duration, i.e. 43% (n = 16) and 48% (n = 24) for the control and intervention group, respectively. Findings from a chi-squared test undertaken found no significant difference between the two groups in terms of duration of labour experienced.

## Mode of delivery

The number of participants who delivered by each mode of delivery, i.e. normal, instrumental and surgical deliveries, is depicted in Table 4.25 and presented in Figure 4.9.

Most participants in both groups experienced normal deliveries, i.e. 67% ($n = 32$) participants in the control group and 74% ($n = 37$) in the intervention group. Findings from a chi-squared test indicated that there was no significant difference between the two groups in terms of mode of delivery.

## Apgar scores of the baby

This is an initial assessment of the general well-being of the newborn routinely carried out at 1 and 5 minutes after all births. There are five assessments, which include heart and respiratory rate, muscle tone, reflexes and colour. Each assessment is scored between 0 and 2 points with a maximum score of 10 points. Higher scores (> 6 points) indicate a healthy baby whereas lower scores (< 6 points) indicate varying degrees of birth asphyxia (Sweet and Tiran 1997).

The number of Apgar scores recorded at 1- and 5-minute assessments are presented in Table 4.26. The range of Apgar scores, for both the control and intervention groups, was between 6 and 10 points at 1 minute and between 7 and 10 points at 5 minutes. Findings from chi-squared tests found no significant difference between the groups in relation to Apgar scores at both 1- and 5-minute assessments.

**Table 4.26** Apgar score at 1 minute and 5 minutes

| Group (1 min) | <7 points | 7 points | 8 points | 9 points | 10 points |
|---|---|---|---|---|---|
| Control ($n = 37$) | 2 (5) | 6 (16) | 23 (63) | 4 (11) | 2 (5) |
| Exercise ($n = 50$) | 2 (4) | 8 (16) | 28 (56) | 8 (16) | 4 (8) |
| | Chi-squared test, $p \geq 0.05$ | | | | |

| Group (5 min) | 7 points | 8 points | 9 points | 10 points | |
|---|---|---|---|---|---|
| Control ($n = 37$) | 2 (5) | 15 (41) | 10 (27) | 10 (27) | |
| Exercise ($n = 50$) | 2 (4) | 10 (20) | 24 (48) | 14 (28) | |
| | Chi-squared test, $p \geq 0.05$ | | | | |

Percentages are given in parentheses.

## Birthweight

A baby weighing 2.5 kg or less is said to be of low birthweight and will need careful paediatric assessment and observation. Low-birthweight babies may be either pre-term, i.e. delivered before 37 completed weeks of pregnancy, or small for gestational age (Sweet and Tiran 1997).

Distribution of babies born within a range of birthweight groups is presented in Table 4.27. Both groups had comparable mean birthweight, i.e. 3.3 (SD 0.4) kg for the control group and 3.4 (0.6) kg for the intervention group.

**Table 4.27** Birthweight

| Group | <2.5 kg | 2.5–2.9 kg | 3.0–3.4 kg | 3.5–3.9 | 4.0–4.4 | 4.5–5.0 kg |
|---|---|---|---|---|---|---|
| Control (n = 37) | 2 (5) | 8 (22) | 10 (27) | 10 (27) | 6 (16) | 1 (3) |
| Exercise (n = 50) | 1 (2) | 12 (24) | 12 (24) | 20 (40) | 3 (6) | 2 (4) |
| | Chi-squared test, $p \geq 0.05$ | | | | | |

Percentages are given in parentheses.

Only 5% (n = 2) of babies in the control group and 2% (n = 1) in the intervention group were identified within the category termed 'low birthweight'. Most of the birthweights were between 3.0 kg and 3.9 kg for both groups. Findings from a chi-squared test indicated no significant difference between the groups in relation to the distribution of birthweight. A two-sample $t$-test was undertaken to investigate the difference in mean birthweight and no significant difference was noted between the groups (Table 4.28).

**Table 4.28** Two-sample $t$-test for birthweight (kg)

| Two-sample $t$-test | n | Mean | SD | SEM |
|---|---|---|---|---|
| Control | 37 | 3.3 | 0.4 | 0.1 |
| Exercise | 50 | 3.4 | 0.6 | 0.1 |

SEM, standard error of the mean; $p \geq 0.05$.

## Maternal or baby complications

The number of complications arising during or after pregnancy, depicted in Table 4.29, indicates that there were no major maternal complications reported in either the control or intervention group during pregnancy. All babies delivered were normal and healthy. However, one subject from the intervention group did require two surgical interventions between birth and 8 weeks after delivery to repair a severely traumatized perineum. Incidentally, this woman gave birth by instrumental delivery to a baby with a birthweight of 5 kg.

**Table 4.29** Maternal or baby complications

| Group | During pregnancy | After pregnancy | Baby |
|---|---|---|---|
| Control (37) | None | None | None |
| Exercise (45) | None | 1 major as a result of perineal trauma | None |

## Pregnancy and birth outcomes (drop-out participants)

Comparison of pregnancy and birth outcomes were repeated with all available information for those participants from each group who failed to complete the study.

The number of participants in relation to length of gestation are presented in Table 4.30. Most participants in both groups were found to deliver between 38 and 40 weeks' gestation, i.e. 74% ($n = 22$) for the control group and 80% ($n = 20$) for the intervention group. No difference was found between the groups in length of gestation, as indicated by a chi-squared test.

The numbers of participants in relation to reported duration of labour are presented in Table 4.31. Most participants experienced labour of between 5 and 8 hours in duration. No significant difference was found between the groups in relation to the duration of labour experienced, as indicated by a chi-squared test.

**Table 4.30** Length of gestation (drop-out participants)

| Group | < 37 weeks | 38–40 weeks | >40 weeks |
|---|---|---|---|
| Control (n = 30) | 4 (13) | 22 (74) | 4 (13) |
| Exercise (n = 25) | 1 (4) | 20 (80) | 4 (16) |
| | Chi-squared test, $p \geq 0.05$ | | |

Percentages are given in parentheses.

**Table 4.31** Duration of labour (drop-out participants)

| Group | <4 hours | 5–8 hours | >8 hours |
|---|---|---|---|
| Control (n = 23) | 6 (26) | 13 (56) | 4 (18) |
| Exercise (n = 25) | 4 (16) | 16 (70) | 5 (22) |
| | Chi-squared test, $p \geq 0.05$ | | |

Percentages are given in parentheses.

The numbers of participants who delivered by the three modes of delivery were comparable. Number and percentage of participants delivering by each of the three delivery modes, i.e. normal, instrumental and surgical deliveries, are presented in Table 4.32. No difference in terms of the mode of delivery was noted between the two groups, as indicated by a chi-squared test.

The range of scores for both groups was between 6 and 9 points at 1 minute and between 7 and 10 points at 5 minutes. The number of Apgar scores at 1-minute and 5-minute assessments is presented in Table 4.33. No difference was noted between the groups in relation to the distribution of Apgar scores at both 1- and 5-minute assessments, as indicated by chi-squared tests.

The range of birthweight was between 2.5 kg and 4.4 kg for the two groups. The distribution of birthweight of babies born to participants who did not complete the study is presented in Table 4.34.

Most of the birthweights for both groups were between 3.0 kg and 3.9 kg, i.e. 67% (n = 20) for the control group and 72% (n = 18) for the intervention group. No difference was found between the groups in relation to the distribution of birthweight as indicated from a chi-squared test undertaken.

**Table 4.32** Mode of delivery (drop-out participants)

| Group | n | Normal (SVD) | Instrumental | Surgical |
|---|---|---|---|---|
| Control | 19 | 7 (36) | 6 (32) | 6 (32) |
| Exercise | 25 | 10 (40) | 10 (40) | 5 (20) |
| | | Chi-squared test, $p \geq 0.05$ | | |

Percentages are given in parentheses.

**Table 4.33** Apgar score at 1 min and 5 min (drop-out participants)

| Group (1 minute) | < 7 points | 7 points | 8 points | 9 points | 10 points |
|---|---|---|---|---|---|
| Control (n = 30) | 3 (10) | 4 (13) | 7 (23) | 16 (53) | 0 (0) |
| Exercise (n = 25) | 2 (8) | 5 (17) | 6 (45) | 12 (28) | 0 (0) |
| | Chi-squared test, $p \geq 0.05$ | | | | |

| Group (5 minute) | 7 points | 8 points | 9 points | 10 points |
|---|---|---|---|---|
| Control (n = 30) | 2 (7) | 4 (13) | 13 (43) | 11 (37) |
| Exercise (n = 25) | 1 (4) | 7 (28) | 5 (20) | 12 (48) |
| | Chi-squared test, $p \geq 0.05$ | | | |

Percentages are given in parentheses.

**Table 4.34** Birthweight (drop-out participants)

| Group | 2.5–2.9 kg | 3.0–3.4 kg | 3.5–3.9 kg | 4.0–4.4 kg |
|---|---|---|---|---|
| Control (n = 29) | 4 (13) | 11 (37) | 9 (30) | 5 (17) |
| Exercise (n = 25) | 5 (20) | 9 (36) | 9 (36) | 4 (16) |
| | Chi-squared test, $p \geq 0.05$ | | | |

Percentages are given in parentheses.

No major maternal or baby complications were reported during or after pregnancy. Details were forwarded to the researcher in relation to two participants allocated to the control group in the antenatal clinic. At this initial appointment, both women were diagnosed by ultrasonography as having a non-continuing pregnancy at 7 and 9 weeks of pregnancy.

In conclusion, both the groups of participants who completed the study and those who dropped out were investigated in relation to the average length of gestation of pregnancy, duration of labour, method of delivery, Apgar scores and birthweight. No significant difference in relation to pregnancy and birth outcomes was noted either between the intervention and control groups or between the groups who completed the study and those who dropped out of the study.

# Physical activity

This section provides details of the findings in relation to the physical activity undertaken by participants during the study. Participants in both groups provided information about physical activity undertaken during and after pregnancy. Activity diaries were maintained by all participants; a summary of levels of activity was obtained at each of the time periods of interest (i.e. early, late and after pregnancy) and a register of attendance was available for participants in the intervention group. Findings are reported in relation to:

- Activity levels in early pregnancy
- Episodes of physical activity
- Types of physical activity
- Drop-out rate of participants
- Frequency of activity.

Levels of activity recorded in early pregnancy and the number of participants, in each classification of activity levels, are shown in Table 4.4 (p. 93). A chi-squared test undertaken on these activity levels indicated that there was no difference among the four different classifications of activity levels between the control and intervention groups in early pregnancy, i.e. inactive, occasionally active, regularly active or very active. Comparisons of activity levels were not followed up during and after pregnancy as a result of insufficient data collected in relation to this particular response.

The participants in both groups recorded episodes of physical activity during and after pregnancy. The method of collecting this information was by the completion of an activity diary followed by subsequent summary of the number of physical activity sessions in early and late pregnancy and after pregnancy, or on completion of the study (see Appendix 14). The intervention group also completed an attendance register at the structured exercise classes (see Appendix 13).

The frequency of the total number of physical activity sessions, including structured exercise sessions, is presented in Table 4.35. The total number of structured exercise classes attended by participants in the intervention group was 1405 sessions, which was 51% of the total physical activity sessions undertaken by participants in the intervention group and 38% of the total physical activity undertaken by participants in both groups. Additional physical activity undertaken by both groups was recorded and classified into categories when the type of activity was identified. The participants in the control group took part in 25% (940) of the total activity sessions (3734) recorded.

Both groups recorded similar types of activities in relation to exercise classes, brisk walking and swimming during the study. There were no recordings of strength training, cycling and yoga type activities in either of the two groups. Two participants, both in the intervention group, reported regular tennis and badminton sessions until the early third trimester of pregnancy. One of these participants reported regular use of the treadmill and Nordic skiing until the third trimester of pregnancy and then again after delivery.

Findings from a chi-squared test, undertaken on additional physical activity sessions, indicated that the intervention group participated in a significantly higher proportion of additional activity sessions than the control group.

Findings from a two-sample $t$-test indicated that there was a significant difference between the two groups in relation to the total average number of physical activity sessions undertaken during and after pregnancy (Table 4.36).

Figure 4.10 presents the total number of physical activity sessions recorded by participants in both groups during the study. Sessions attended by the control group indicated that a number of participants

**Table 4.35** Frequency of the total number of physical activity sessions including structured exercise sessions

| Group | Structured exercise classes | Other classes, e.g. aerobic or aquanatal | Brisk walk | Swim | Golf or tennis | Treadmill or Nordic ski | Total number |
|---|---|---|---|---|---|---|---|
| Control (n = 48) | 0 (0) | 425 (45) | 300 (32) | 215 (23) | 0 (0) | 0 (0) | 940 |
| Exercise (n = 75) | 1405 (51) | 300 (11) | 275 (10) | 450 (17) | 284 (10) | 80 (1) | 2794 |
| | | Chi-squared test, p < 0.001 | | | | | |
| Total | 1405 (38) | 725 (20) | 575 (16) | 665 (18) | 180 (6) | 80 (2) | 3734 |

Percentages are given in parentheses.

**Table 4.36** Two-sample *t*-test for physical activity sessions

| Total number of sessions | n | Mean | SD | SEM |
|---|---|---|---|---|
| Control | 48 | 18.7 | 48.5 | 6.9 |
| Exercise | 50 | 55.6 | 26.8 | 3.9 |

Two-sample t-test for total number of sessions, $p < 0.0001$
Range for control group: 0–120 sessions
Range for intervention group: 0–200 sessions

Percentages are given in parentheses.

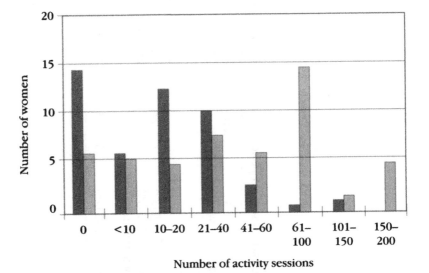

**Figure 4.10** The total number of physical activity sessions attended by participants during the study. ☐ Exercise group; ■ Control group.

remained active during and after pregnancy. However, it can be seen from Figure 4.10 that most of these participants took part in fewer than a total of 60 sessions during the course of the study, with only a few undertaking between 61 and 150 sessions.

The relationship between the frequency of physical activity undertaken during the study and the psychological indicators of coping assets (positive psychological well-being), coping deficits (negative psychological well-being) and physical well-being after pregnancy was investigated by correlation analyses using Pearson's product–moment coefficient of correlations. The findings are presented in Table 4.37.

There was no significant relationship found between the frequency of reported physical activity and the responses of the three psychological indicators after pregnancy.

**Table 4.37** Correlation coefficients for the relationship between frequency of physical activity and psychological indicators

| Psychological indicators | Correlation coefficient | |
| --- | --- | --- |
| Coping assets (positive psychological well-being) | $r = 0.21$ | $p = 0.15$ |
| Coping deficits (negative psychological well-being) | $r = -0.14$ | $p = 0.33$ |
| Perceptions of physical well-being | $r = 0.16$ | $p = 0.26$ |

Findings concluded that participants in the intervention group did participate in a significantly higher number of physical activity sessions than the participants in the control group. There was no significant relationship between the frequency of physical activity and the psychological indicators of coping assets (positive psychological well-being), coping deficits (negative psychological well-being) and perceptions of physical well-being after pregnancy.

## Drop-out from the study

The timing and number of participants in each group who dropped out during the study are presented in Table 4.38. A total of 38% ($n = 59$) of the participants dropped out of the study, of whom 36% ($n = 39$) were from the control group and 39% ($n = 32$) from the intervention group.

Most of the participants who dropped out of the study (32%; $n = 49$) did so between recruitment and 20 weeks' gestation, i.e. 29% ($n = 22$) from the control group and 33% ($n = 27$) from the intervention group. Only a few questionnaires were returned during this stage and, as a result, this information was not available for inclusion within the study. Thereafter, the number of participants who dropped out of the study, i.e. control 7% ($n = 5$), intervention group 6% ($n = 5$), did so at various times between 24 and 32 weeks' gestation. The remaining participants

**Table 4.38** The timing and number of participants who dropped out of the study

| Group | n | Number (%) and weeks of drop-out participants from the study | | | | |
| --- | --- | --- | --- | --- | --- | --- |
| | | 12–20 weeks | 24 weeks | 28 weeks | 32 weeks | Completed |
| Control | 75 | 22 (29) | 2 (3) | 1 (1) | 2 (3) | 48 (64) |
| Exercise | 82 | 27 (33) | 1 (1) | 2 (2.5) | 2 (2.5) | 50 (61) |
| | | Chi-squared test, $p = (0.05)$ | | | | |
| Total n (%) | 157 | 49 (32) | | 10 (6) | | 98 (62) |
| | | Total number of drop-out participants from the study = 59 (38) | | | | |

completed the study, i.e. 64% ($n$ = 48) in the control group and 61% ($n$ = 50) in the intervention group. Findings from a chi-squared test indicated that there was no significant difference between the groups in relation to the participants who dropped out of the study in the initial stages, during the study and those participants who completed the study.

The age group of participants who dropped out of the study is presented in Table 4.39. Most participants in both groups were aged between 26 and 30 years, i.e. 48% ($n$ = 13) for the control group and 44% ($n$ = 14) for the intervention group. No significant difference was found between the groups in relation to age group, as indicated by a chi-squared test.

Relationship status and employment status of participants who dropped out of the study are presented in Table 4.40. In both groups, most of the participants who dropped out were married and in employment. In the control group, 44% ($n$ = 12) of participants were married and 88% were in employment. In comparison, 63% ($n$ = 20) of the participants in the intervention group were married and 78% ($n$ = 25) were in employment.

**Table 4.39** Age group of participants who dropped out of the study

| Group | < 20 years | 21–25 years | 26–30 years | 31–35 years | > 35 years |
|---|---|---|---|---|---|
| Control (n = 27) | 2 (7) | 4 (16) | 13 (48) | 6 (22) | 2 (7) |
| Exercise (n = 32) | 3 (9) | 5 (16) | 14 (44) | 9 (28) | 1 (3) |
| | Chi-squared test, $p \geq 0.05$ | | | | |

Percentages are given in parentheses.

**Table 4.40** Relationship and employment status of participants who dropped out of the study

| Group | Relationship status | | | Employment status | | |
|---|---|---|---|---|---|---|
| | Married | Partner | Single | Employed | Unemployed | Student |
| Control (n = 27) | 12 (44) | 10 (37) | 5 (19) | 24 (89) | 3 (11) | 0 |
| Exercise (n = 32) | 20 (63) | 9 (28) | 3 (9) | 25 (78) | 7 (22) | 0 |
| | Chi-squared test, $p \geq 0.05$ | | | Chi-squared test, $p \geq 0.05$ | | |

Percentages are given in parentheses.

Findings from chi-squared tests indicated that there was no significant difference between the two groups in relation to relationship status and employment status of the participants who dropped out of the study.

Data for the activity levels in early pregnancy were available only from participants who dropped out of this study if this information was provided. This information is presented in Table 4.41. Activity levels of the drop-outs were comparable between the two groups and no significant difference was indicated from a chi-squared test.

These findings indicate that most participants in both groups who failed to complete the study were married, employed and aged between 26 and 30 years of age.

Reasons for leaving the study were not given in most cases, especially for those participants who failed to complete the initial questionnaire after recruitment, i.e. excluding the two participants from the control group who experienced a non-continuing pregnancy before 10 weeks' gestation. The participants in the intervention group offered a few reasons. These included:

> It was too tiring after work to come to the exercise class.
> I just do not have the energy.
> It was too far to travel to the hospital.

Only anecdotal information was obtained in relation to the reason for any of the participants in the control group failing to continue with the study. This information included comments about specific participants who had wanted to exercise and preferred to be participants in the intervention group. Another reason offered suggested that some participants thought that they were automatically out of the study because they did not complete or return the questionnaire at the appropriate time.

**Table 4.41** Activity levels of participants who dropped out during the study

| Group | Classification of activity levels at time of recruitment | | | |
| --- | --- | --- | --- | --- |
| | Inactive | Occasionally active | Regularly active | Very active |
| Control (n = 5) | 2 (40) | 1 (20) | 1 (20) | 1 (20) |
| Exercise (n = 5) | 1 (20) | 1 (20) | 1 (20) | 2 (40) |
| | Chi–squared test, $p \geq 0.05$ | | | |

Percentages are given in parentheses.

**Limitations of the study**

The present study was a randomized controlled study of healthy participants during and after their first pregnancy. The control group of participants continued with the existing antenatal preparation for pregnancy, childbirth and the transition to motherhood. In addition, the intervention group participated in a structured antenatal and postnatal exercise programme. Information was collected in early pregnancy (12–16 weeks), late pregnancy (36–40 weeks) and after pregnancy (12–16 weeks).

The study was long in duration and followed participants during a significant time of change in their lives. This included the physiological and psychological changes of pregnancy and childbirth, changing lifestyles and changing roles, and new responsibilities. These were challenges that faced not only the participants but also the researcher. This was a difficult task but on the whole most participants in both groups completed the study.

The return of questionnaires was slow at times and many participants had to be prompted. This mainly related to some of the participants in the control group. The same few participants continued to complete the questionnaires inaccurately. This was a particular problem after the birth of the baby. It was not possible to investigate how participants described themselves in relation to the levels of activity during the study. This information was available in early pregnancy but was omitted from most of the returned questionnaires as a result of the lack of clarity in the design of the questionnaire.

The attendance record maintained at the exercise class was reliable, giving accurate information about the frequency of attendance for the participants in the intervention group. In addition, most of these participants also maintained accurate activity diaries of additional activities. However, the accuracy of some of the activity diaries maintained by participants in the control group and some in the intervention group remains uncertain. If anything, the researcher suspected that more physical activity was performed than was recorded.

Often the subjective information about the pregnancy and birth details did not correspond with the information on the birth register. This discrepancy could be quite marked at times, especially in relation to the duration of labour. The researcher tended to rely on the information available from the birth register.

On several occasions, women arrived at the structured exercise class who were not in the study. This was a dilemma for the researcher who made alternative exercise arrangements for them.

On a positive note, many women in the postnatal period continued to attend the class after they had completed the study. This proved to be a problem, especially as new participants were being recruited. The researcher used the postnatal reunion as an opportunity to say thank you to these participants. Alternative exercise arrangements were made for these participants.

A word of warning to any reader who may intend to take exercise classes involving postnatal mothers and babies. Ensure that you have friends or helpers who can assist with the babies when the new mother is exercising. Also, design the programme to allow the new mother to breast-feed her baby, if necessary.

# Conclusion

This chapter has provided details of statistical analyses and findings of the present study, in relation to the recruitment and retention of the participants, demographic details, psychological indicators of interest, pregnancy and birth outcomes, and physical activity details.

In summary, no differences were noted between the groups in relation to:

- Demographic details including age, marital and employment status
- Levels of activity reported in early pregnancy
- Pregnancy outcomes in relation to the length of pregnancy, duration of labour and type of delivery, for both those participants who completed and those who did not complete the study
- Birth outcomes in relation to birthweight and Apgar score of babies at 1 and 5 minutes after birth, for babies born to both those participants who completed and those who did not complete the study
- Postnatal emotional well-being/depression
- Maternal and neonatal complications experienced.

Significant differences were found between the groups in relation to the number of episodes of exercise undertaken during and after pregnancy, psychological indicators including perception of coping assets (positive psychological well-being), coping deficits (negative psychological well-being), physical well-being, somatic symptoms experienced, body image, and attitudes to marital relationships, sex and to pregnancy and the baby:

- The participants in the intervention group took part in a significantly higher number of episodes of physical activity than the participants in the control group.

- No significant relationship was found between the frequency of physical activity and the psychological indicators of positive and negative psychological well-being after pregnancy.
- Significant differences were found between the groups in relation to perceptions of coping assets (positive psychological well-being) and coping deficits (negative psychological well-being), physical well-being, somatic symptoms experienced, body image, and in the attitudes to marital relationships, sex and to pregnancy and baby. Participants in the intervention group tended to protect or experience a delay in the reduction of these indicators during and after pregnancy. This was in contrast to the participants in the control group who had significant reductions over the same period of time.

The next chapter discusses these findings and integrates them with the current literature.

# Chapter 5
# Discussion

This chapter discusses the findings of the study in relation to meeting its aims. The findings are integrated with the current literature available in the area of interest. The discussion encompasses three separate but related themes. The first section focuses on the psychological indicators of well-being. Within this section, there is a general overview of the findings presented, followed by a general discussion of the possible influencing factors. Thereafter, each psychological indicator is discussed separately. Any issues previously discussed are highlighted if they have a particular significance to the current issue. The second section discusses the findings related to pregnancy and birth outcomes, and the findings are integrated within the findings from the current literature. Discussion focuses on the physical activity of the participants and adherence to the study in the third section. Finally, a summary of the main discussion points and their relevance to findings from the current literature are presented.

## Psychological indicators

The findings of this study suggest that participants who took regular physical activity, maintained their early pregnancy levels of psychological well-being during and after pregnancy; these were noted to deteriorate in the control participants. Psychological indicators of well-being encompassed how women felt about themselves and their bodies, how well they felt they could cope, and their attitudes to marital relationships, sex, and to pregnancy and the baby.

In early pregnancy, no significant differences were found between participants in the control group and intervention group in relation to seven of the eight psychological indicators of well-being that are of interest. These included levels in perceptions of: coping assets (positive psychological well-being), coping deficits (negative psychological well-being), physical well-being, somatic symptoms experienced, and attitudes to marital relationships, pregnancy and sex. As a result of random allocation of the participants to the two groups, it was anticipated that baseline measures on all psychological indicators of well-being would be comparable at the start of the study before any intervention has occurred. This randomization process should have controlled for any confounding bias and ensured that all participants had an equal chance of being allocated to either of the two groups. However, in contrast to the other psychological indicators of well-being, participants in the control group entered the study with small but significantly higher perceptions of body image than the participants in the intervention group. This finding is difficult to explain, especially as the other psychological indicators of well-being were comparable between the groups at this initial stage. As this was an isolated finding, it can be explained by attributing it to a chance occurrence.

Significant differences were noted between the two groups in all the psychological indicators of well-being investigated. These significant differences were noted from early pregnancy until 4 months after delivery. Subjects who participated in regular physical activity tended to maintain their perceptions in terms of how well they felt that they could cope, physical well-being, somatic symptoms experienced, body image, and attitudes to sex and marital relationships during and after pregnancy. In contrast, the participants in the control group, during the same period, reported significant reductions in their perceptions of how well they felt that they could cope, physical well-being, somatic symptoms experienced and body image. These psychological indicators of well-being for the participants in the control group did tend to improve after pregnancy but had not yet returned to early pregnancy levels by 4 months after delivery.

In relation to perceptions of coping deficits (negative psychological well-being), participants in the control group reported a significant increase in these perceptions, which was further evidence of an inability to cope during this period. After delivery, participants in both groups showed positive increase in their attitudes to the baby, but levels for participants in the control group had not reached the levels observed in early pregnancy. These findings strongly suggested that participation in regular physical activity was associated with a beneficial protection or delay in a reduction of psychological well-being during and after pregnancy.

Pregnancy is an emotional and vulnerable time for women. In general, it is normally expected for women to have a reduction in psychological well-being during pregnancy. This is a typical feature of pregnancy and does not imply abnormal or poor psychological adjustment (Niven 1992). During this life event, women have to cope with physical and physiological changes, physical discomforts, lifestyle changes and other social factors (Artal Mittlemark et al. 1991b). Therefore, maintenance or delay in any deterioration of psychological well-being during pregnancy can only be beneficial.

The way in which a woman reacts to the profound body and social changes during pregnancy are influenced to a large extent by her personality, her lifestyle, her relationship with her partner and her feelings about herself, pregnancy and baby, and her level of physical fitness (Artal Mittlemark et al. 1991b; Wells 1991). When this is considered, it is possible that regular physical activity influenced several of these factors, which in turn enabled participants to experience pregnancy more positively and subsequently supported their transition to motherhood.

## Influencing factors

In the present study, the psychological benefit gained by the participants in the intervention group might have been influenced directly by the exercise itself or indirectly by other factors, including psychosocial support, group interaction and participation in a research study.

## Benefits of exercise

First, it is generally accepted that there are both physical and psychological benefits to be gained by regular exercise. These include improved stamina, agility and muscular strength, positive feelings of well-being and feelings of being in control (Allied Dunbar National Fitness Survey 1992; Bouchard and Stephens 1993). Regular participation in physical activity would give participants the opportunity to maintain or improve physical fitness, and improve posture and body awareness and muscle tone.

The participants in the intervention group did take part in significantly more sessions of physical activity than the participants in the control group. There was no significant relationship between the frequency of physical activity and the responses of psychological indicators after pregnancy. This suggests that other factors related to the exercise may be responsible for the psychological well-being rather than the frequency of the physical activity. Other factors directly associated with the activity may include the type, duration and intensity of the activity.

Indirect factors associated with the psychological benefits experienced may be related to an interaction of exercise with other factors, such as social interaction and factors to be discussed in this section. It does remain a strong possibility that exercise participation may directly influence the psychological well-being experienced by the participants in the intervention group, although other factors are still a possibility and should be given due consideration.

## Psychosocial support

Other equally important factors may be indirect and include the possible benefit gained from social interaction and planned recreational time for the participants at the exercise class. Psychosocial support is a key component in the psychological care of women during pregnancy (Hirst et al. 1998) and has a positive influence on their mental health (Oakley 1992; Wheatley 1998). Pregnant women regard good quality support as including good interpersonal skills within a facilitative environment (Oakley 1992). Women who received good support reported significantly enhanced emotional well-being (Oakley 1992; Wheatley 1998), more confidence and self-reliance (Hirst et al. 1998). Women who exercised regularly during pregnancy are reported to experience psychological and social benefits (Lee 1996).

In the present study, the social interaction provided by the class situation may have given the participants the opportunity to have a mutual sharing of pregnancy-related worries and concerns with their peers. This may have contributed to reduced anxiety, improved feelings of security and self-worth which, in turn, prevented the reduction in psychological indicators of well-being normally experienced by women during pregnancy. The social support experienced by participants attending the exercise class may have positively influenced psychological well-being.

Both participation in the study and feeling a part of a group may also have contributed to participants in the valued intervention group feeling. Wheatley (1998) suggests that women who feel accepted within a group and gain positive feedback from the interaction with their peers experience reduced anxiety, reduced antenatal and postnatal depression, increased self-esteem and increased confidence. Participation in the exercise programme itself may have served as a form of distraction for participants, by diverting their thoughts and feelings about themselves and their bodily functions.

The interaction with the exercise instructor was also an important factor to consider. A positive interaction between the instructor and the participants in the exercise class may have influenced some of them. Possible contributing factors may include the gain of a positive attitude towards exercise and positive reinforcement for attendance at the class, general acceptance within the group, motivation and enthusiasm, and the possible development of a mutual friendship. The participants may also have been more enthusiastic about completing the questionnaires, resulting in a more prompt response to the requests for information than that experienced by the participants in the control group.

The control participants continued with the existing antenatal preparation for pregnancy and childbirth, and therefore had opportunities for physical activity and social support through the facilities offered. The normal reduction in psychological well-being experienced by these participants during the course of the study was significantly higher than for the participants in the intervention group. Possible factors contributing to these findings include a significantly reduced number of episodes of activity undertaken and therefore less opportunity to gain the direct and indirect benefits of physical activity.

Participants allocated to the control group may have preferred to be in the intervention group. This could make them feel less inclined to be involved in the research study. The limited direct contact with the researcher during the course of the study may have been a negative factor. Completed information was always more difficult to obtain from the participants in the control group. One or more of these factors may have contributed to participants in the control group having reduced enthusiasm, willingness and motivation to complete the questionnaires, provide valid information about their feelings and attitudes, and offer information willingly.

## Perceptions of coping assets and deficits

Pregnancy may have a negative influence on the emotional and psychological well-being of women (Artal and Artal Mittlemark 1991). The literature has suggested that pregnant women experience a range of emotional and psychological changes. Anxiety levels are reported to increase as pregnancy progresses (Green 1990a). Niven (1992) recommends that maternal anxiety should be reduced to improve emotional and psychological well-being.

The findings from the present study indicate significant differences between the two groups in relation to how participants perceived that they could cope during and after pregnancy. The participants in the control group had a significant decrease in their perceived ability to cope during and after pregnancy and a significant increase in perceived coping deficits (negative psychological well-being). In contrast, the participants in the intervention group tended to maintain their early pregnancy levels on both these indicators of psychological well-being during the same period.

These findings support the existing literature pertaining to the non-pregnant population, which suggests that exercise contributes to achieving optimal psychological well-being. Physical activity has been positively associated with general well-being (Plummer and Koh 1987; Stephens 1988; Crammer et al. 1991). Other positive associations include lower levels of anxiety (Roth and Holmes 1987; Moses et al. 1989; Steptoe et al. 1989), improved coping abilities and reduced tension (Morgan 1985).

Other researchers have used the psychological indicators of perceived coping assets, coping deficits and well-being in studies of physical activity with the general population. Steptoe et al. (1989) report a significant increase in coping assets and a significant decrease in coping deficits with normal healthy individuals over a training period. In this present study, the intervention group maintained early pregnancy levels in coping assets (positive psychological well-being) and coping deficits (negative psychological well-being) during and after pregnancy. This was in contrast to the control group who had significant reductions in coping assets (positive psychological well-being) and significant increases in coping deficits (negative psychological well-being) during the same period. It was not possible to make a comparison of the baseline response to these psychological indicators with participants in the current study because Steptoe et al. (1989) report only the changes in the psychological indicators during the training period.

Loughlan (1995) studied healthy middle-aged participants taking part in a health-related physical activity study over a period of 6 months. He reported a significant improvement in coping deficits over this period. In the present study, the intervention group had similar findings in coping assets (positive psychological well-being) and physical well-being, but this group did not show any significant improvements in coping deficits (negative psychological well-being), which were actually maintained during the study. It was interesting to note that, in the study by Loughlan (1995), the participants reported similar levels in both coping assets and physical well-being to the early pregnancy levels of participants in the present study. However, in the present study the early pregnancy levels of coping deficits (negative psychological well-being) tended to be more positive than the commencement levels of participants in the study conducted by Loughlan (1995). The participants and duration of the intervention should be considered when comparing both studies. The present study had healthy young participants ($n$ = 98) from early pregnancy until 4 months after delivery of the baby whereas, in contrast, the other study was of shorter duration and involved healthy, middle-aged male and female participants. Although limited, comparison with studies of the general population was informative because findings in the present study were similar to the psychological indicators of well-being in other populations. As there was no available literature of similar studies during pregnancy, it was not possible to make comparisons of the psychological indicators of other participants during and after pregnancy.

There is very little available scientific information about the psychological aspects of exercise in pregnancy. There was no evidence of any relationship between the total physical activity undertaken and the psychological indicators of coping assets (positive psychological well-being), coping deficits (negative psychological well-being) and physical well-being. The present findings do suggest that regular physical activity maintains or delays the reduction in psychological well-being normally experienced during pregnancy. There is only agreement with the findings of this present study and other similar studies, in that participants who exercised regularly had significantly higher levels of psychological well-being when compared with sedentary individuals or participants in control groups. Therefore, the present findings offer support only to the general trend found in the limited number of studies that report on the psychological benefits of exercise during pregnancy. There was no evidence of any improvements on early pregnancy levels for psychological indicators of well-being within this study. In contrast, other researchers suggest that exercise during pregnancy enhances a sense of well-being, increases total self-esteem (Sibley et al. 1981; Wallace et al. 1986; Wolfe et al. 1989a, b; Koniak-Griffin 1994) and reduces tension (Hall and Kaufmann 1987).

Findings from all of these previous studies suggest positive psychological benefits from the participation in exercise during pregnancy. However, one main disadvantage attributed to many of these studies has been the use of self-selected participants, which detracts from the credibility of the findings and limits their application. This recognized limitation in research design was considered during the planning of the present study. Randomization of participants to the two groups was used in an attempt to address this disadvantage within this study. It is hoped that the significantly positive psychological well-being experienced by participants in the intervention group during and after pregnancy can be generalized to other healthy primigravid women.

The participants in the intervention group did maintain perceptions of coping assets (positive psychological well-being) and coping deficits (negative psychological well-being), in contrast to a deterioration of these perceptions for the participants in the control group.

There is a strong possibility that participation in regular exercise contributed to these findings, but other factors such as psychosocial support and group interaction may have contributed and need to be recognized as a possible influencing factor.

## Perceptions of physical well-being and somatic symptoms

Women experience increased experiences of somatic conditions during pregnancy. This may be caused by the physiological adaptations of pregnancy. Other factors such as physical and psychological concerns of women may exacerbate these conditions as pregnancy approaches labour and delivery of the baby (Niven 1992). Increased experience of the symptoms of pregnancy is associated with negative attitudes towards pregnancy (Raphael-Leff 1991).

Those who participated in regular physical activity within this study maintained their perceptions of physical well-being during and after pregnancy when compared with control participants. Regular physical activity undoubtedly contributes to improved stamina and physical well-being and this would benefit women during pregnancy and childbirth (Artal Mittlemark et al. 1991b; Riemann and Kanstrup-Hansen 2000).

Findings from the present study indicate that participants in the intervention group maintained their perception of the somatic symptoms experienced during and after pregnancy. This was in contrast to significantly negative perceptions in somatic symptoms experienced during pregnancy by the control participants. Limited literature is available of similar studies during pregnancy to enable comparisons of research findings. However, other researchers suggest that women who exercise regularly during pregnancy report significant increase in vigour (Koltyn and Schultes 1997), significantly lower incidence of physical symptoms (Wallace et al. 1986), decrease in physical discomforts during pregnancy (Horns et al. 1996) and reductions in physical complaints after childbirth (Hall and Kaufmann 1987). Many of these studies included self-selected participants, which limited the application of findings to only active pregnant participants. The present study investigated the perceptions of physical well-being and somatic symptoms experienced as opposed to the frequency and measurement of physical discomforts. However, the present findings give support to the general trend found in other studies that women who exercise during and after pregnancy have significantly more positive levels in relation to physical well-being and somatic symptoms experienced.

There is a strong possibility that participation in the physical activity may have directly influenced these findings. Improved muscular strength gained from regular exercise would be beneficial to pregnant women. This would improve posture and prevent back pain, improve mobility, and develop body awareness to facilitate the physical changes brought about by pregnancy. Research findings report that women who exercise regularly do experience improved posture and mobility (Lee 1996). There is a strong possibility that participation in a regular exercise programme influenced these findings as a result of the physical benefits gained from exercise participation. Other influencing factors such as psychosocial support also need to be acknowledged.

## Perceptions of body image

Pregnancy can be viewed as being an unattractive condition, and a reduction in perceptions of body image occurs during this time (Raphael-Leff 1991). Strang and Sullivan (1985) suggest that women are dissatisfied with the changing shape of the body as pregnancy progresses and this dissatisfaction can be even more profound in new mothers (Strang and Sullivan 1985). However, anecdotal information suggests that women are more positive about their bodies after delivery.

In the present study, participants in the control group tended to have significantly more negative perceptions of body image during and after pregnancy despite having significantly higher and more positive perceptions than the participants in the intervention group on commencement of the study. This was in contrast to maintenance of perceptions of body image during and after pregnancy for the participants in the intervention group during the same period.

There is limited available literature of similar studies of exercise and related body image during pregnancy. Slavin et al. (1988) concludes that regular exercise during pregnancy allows women to have control over their bodies at a time of profound bodily changes. It is suggested that exercise may have a positive role to play in the way pregnant women feel about themselves, their femaleness and their bodies (Artal and Artal Mittlemark 1991).

One of the major contributing factors to the critical nature of the postnatal period is the changing body shape and appearance (Price 1993b). Therefore, the enhanced perception of body image experienced by participants who participated in regular physical activity would, no doubt, have contributed to the maintenance of early pregnancy levels of psychological well-being reported during and after pregnancy.

The maintenance in perceptions of body image experienced by the participants who exercised during this study may have been influenced by the interaction of other psychological variables, including the perceptions of physical well-being and the ability to cope (positive psychological well-being). Possible factors may have, to some extent, influenced these perceptions through either direct or indirect gain from the participation in regular physical activity. Factors directly gained from exercise participation included improved muscle tone and physical fitness, and improved feelings of physical and psychological well-being (ADNFS 1992; Bouchard et al. 1994).

Participants in the intervention group maintained their perceptions of body image during pregnancy in comparison to deterioration in perceptions of body image experienced by participants in the control group. Participation in a regular exercise programme may have been a strong influencing factor as participants gained the reported physical and psychological benefits of exercise. Other factors such as psycho-social support may have influenced these findings.

### Attitudes to marital relationships, sex and pregnancy/baby

Pregnancy and new parenting occur within a relatively short time frame. During this time, factors influencing relationships include a variety of interpersonal, social, cultural and physical challenges. All of these factors need to be taken into consideration when studying an individual's sexual identity and shared relationships (Raphael-Leff 1991; Niven 1992). Pregnancy causes major changes in marital and cohabiting relationships, and it is proposed that the woman's experience of her body may extend to affect feelings of sex and postpartum relationships (Price 1993b).

Findings from this present study were difficult to interpret within this very personal and complex situation. There are many psychological and social factors, which may contribute to the interaction of marital relationships and sex (Scott-Heyes 1984; Watson et al. 1984; Raphael-Leff 1991). Significant differences were found between the participants in the two groups in relation to their attitudes to marital relationships and sex during and after pregnancy. No differences were noted in the participants in the intervention group during and after pregnancy. In contrast, the participants in the control group had significant negative reductions in their attitudes to marital relationships and sex during the same period, which was more marked for the attitudes to sex after delivery of the baby. Comparison of these findings with other similar studies was not possible as a result of a lack of available literature in this field.

In the present study, the protection of early pregnancy levels of psychological well-being experienced by participants in the intervention group, in comparison to that of the control participants, may have influenced the more positive attitudes to marital relationships and sex. This influence or interaction may have been in terms of more positive perceptions of how well they could cope, physical well-being, somatic symptoms experienced and body image. Psychological well-being may have better prepared participants in the intervention group to meet and overcome any challenges or situations occurring within their marital relationships.

There is general agreement in the literature that a woman's level of sexual interest changes during pregnancy and remains altered for weeks or months after the birth (Niven 1992; Barclay et al. 1994). Interpretation of the findings of the present study, in terms of attitudes to marital relationships and sex, was fraught by a number of diverse contributing factors such as social, cultural and lifestyle implications. However, it was possible that exercise directly or indirectly influenced the more positive attitudes noted in the participants in the intervention group, especially in relation to maintaining the attitude to sex in the postnatal period. An interaction of these influencing factors may have included more positive perceptions of body image, physical and emotional well-being, somatic symptoms experienced and the ability to cope, in addition to the physical benefits gained through participating in regular exercise. Any positive interaction of these factors may have subsequently influenced more positive attitudes to marital relationships and sexual interest. There is a complex interaction between a couple and the changes in the participant's sexual interest. However, the potential synergism of sexual interest and sexual behaviour within a relationship is poorly understood, especially in relation to pregnancy.

After delivery of the baby, participants in both groups had positive and significant increases in attitudes to the baby, with participants in the control group not yet returning to early pregnancy levels and those in the intervention group exceeding their early pregnancy levels. Findings from the participants in the control group follow the normal trend experienced by pregnant participants, who become more positive in their attitudes once the fears and anxieties related to the birth process are removed. The higher levels experienced in attitudes to pregnancy by the participants in the intervention group may be the result of the positive influence of exercise or interrelated factors in the protection of psychological well-being during pregnancy.

There is a strong possibility that participation in a regular exercise programme enables participants in the intervention group to gain the psychological benefits of exercise. These benefits may have influenced the participants in the intervention group to maintain psychological well-being, which, in turn, influenced their attitudes towards themselves, pregnancy and relationships.

In the present study, no significant difference was found between the participants in both groups in terms of postnatal emotional well-being and depression. All participants experienced positive emotional well-being with no evidence of any tendency towards depressive states. However, more positive emotional well-being was observed for participants in the intervention group when compared with participants in the control group. More positive psychological well-being experienced during pregnancy by participants in the intervention group may influence postnatal emotional well-being. In contrast, the significant deterioration in the psychological well-being experienced during pregnancy by participants in the control group may have influenced their levels of postnatal emotional well-being.

In summary, significant differences were noted between the two groups in all the psychological indicators of well-being investigated. These significant differences were noted from early pregnancy until 4 months after delivery. Participants in the intervention group tended to maintain their perceptions in terms of how well they felt that they could cope, physical well-being, somatic symptoms experienced, body image, and attitudes to sex and marital relationships during and after pregnancy. In contrast, the participants in the control group, during the same period, reported significant reductions in their perceptions of how well they felt that they could cope, physical well-being, somatic symptoms experienced and body image. These psychological indicators of well-being for the participants in the control group did tend to improve after pregnancy but had not yet returned to early pregnancy levels by 4 months after delivery.

The findings from the current study, in relation to psychological indicators of well-being, will allow practitioners involved with the care of pregnant women (i.e. midwives and general practitioners) to recommend regular participation in physical activity during pregnancy. This will enable women to maintain psychological and emotional well-being and self-image during and after pregnancy. Childbirth is a recognized critical and emotional event in women's lives, when it is important that physical and psychological well-being is either maintained or enhanced to make this experience as positive as possible for them.

## Pregnancy and birth outcomes

The complex interaction between the physiological adaptation to exercise and pregnancy suggests that these adaptations should impact on each other. Based on the published literature to date, it has not been possible to conclude in any scientific way whether maternal exercise influences pregnancy and birth outcomes.

Findings from this present study found no difference between the control group and intervention group in relation to pregnancy and birth outcomes. This included the length of pregnancy, duration of labour, mode of delivery, birthweight, Apgar scores of babies, and maternal and neonatal complications experienced.

## Pregnancy outcomes

The effect of physical activity during pregnancy on pre-term delivery and fetal growth is a controversial issue. Health professionals and the women themselves have concerns that regular physical activity may result in pre-term delivery. Many possible factors may contribute to the onset of uterine activity, including obstetric and medical considerations, social and environmental factors, and lifestyle factors. Pre-term delivery remains one of the most important factors that affect infant mortality and morbidity. There is no doubt that pre-term labour and delivery may compromise the fetus and have possible adverse effects on the newborn.

There is the concern that, theoretically, uterine activity may be stimulated by the increase in circulating catecholamines with exercise (Gorski 1985). Careful consideration is given to this issue, but, to date, there is no evidence to support this concern within the findings of current research studies (Clapp 2000; Riemann and Kanstrup-Hansen 2000).

In the present study, no significant difference was found between the groups in terms of the length of gestation at delivery. These findings support much of the available literature which indicates that regular exercise is not associated with the incidence of pre-term labour or has an adverse early pregnancy outcome (Pomerance et al. 1974; Veille et al. 1985; Clapp 1989, 1990; Beckmann and Beckmann 1990; Botkin and Driscoll 1991; Zeanah and Schlosser 1993).

In general, the present findings suggest that physical activity did not have any effect on the shortening of gestation of pregnancy. However, when comparing and contrasting these findings with those from other studies, it is important to consider that participants in the current study were 'low-risk' primigravidae who did not experience any medical or obstetric conditions that may have contributed to pre-term delivery.

Many women believe that, if they exercise during pregnancy, they will become more fit and this will result in an easier labour and delivery. Riemann and Kanstrup Hansen (2000) suggest that women in labour would benefit from being physically fit. It would be logical to expect labour to be facilitated as a result of physical conditioning as a result of enhanced maternal working capacity and improved function of specific muscles used in labour.

No significant difference was found in the current study between the two groups of participants in terms of the total duration of labour and mode of delivery. Most participants in both groups had normal deliveries at term. Subjective experiences about the experience of labour were not investigated. No maternal, fetal or neonatal complications were reported during pregnancy or labour for the women participating in the study. There was one incident of a woman from the intervention group who required two episodes of surgical intervention within the first 6 weeks after delivery. This was caused by severe trauma to the perineum during the instrumental delivery of a baby with a birthweight of 5 kg.

Other research has also focused on clinical issues related to the outcome of the labour and delivery. Existing studies used the duration of the stages of labour as an indication of the difficulty of labour. The indication that the difficulty of labour is related to the duration of the stages of labour is questionable, especially in modern-day obstetric practice. However, women do perceive this to be an indication of how well they will cope with labour. Generally, women associate short labour with a relatively easy labour and more difficult labours with a longer duration of labour.

Research findings in the relationship of exercise and the positive outcomes for mother and baby are of interest to researchers. Numerous studies have investigated the effect that exercise has on labour and delivery, resulting in a variety of findings. Some findings indicate that there is no difference in the duration of labour between physically active and sedentary women (Kupla et al. 1987; Rose et al. 1991; Lee 1996; Kardel and Kase 1998). The present study found no difference in the duration of labour and lends support to studies with similar findings.

Findings from other studies indicate that women who exercise during pregnancy report significantly shorter time in the active second stage of labour compared with sedentary women (Hall and Kaufmann 1987; Botkin and Driscoll 1991; Zeanah and Schlosser 1993). Findings from the study by Kupla et al. (1987) found no differences in the duration of labour between multigravid participants, but did report that primigravid participants who exercised had a significantly shorter active stage of labour than sedentary women. This is in contrast to the present findings where primigravid participants were investigated.

This present study investigated the total time of labour from onset until delivery of the baby and the timing of different stages of labour was not identified. This made comparison with these other studies difficult because the duration of the two stages of labour was reported and not the summation of findings about the duration of labour.

No differences were found, in the present study, in the type of delivery and incidence of obstetric complications. These findings agree with the findings of other researchers (Kupla et al. 1987; Lee 1996; Kardel and Kase 1998). In contrast, other researchers noted a significant reduction in the incidence of obstetric complications and interventions with women who exercise during pregnancy (Clapp 1990; Botkin and Driscoll 1991; Zeanah and Schlosser 1993; Wang and Apgar 1998) and in the incidence of surgical deliveries (Hall and Kaufmann 1987).

However, labour and delivery are both very complex processes involving many factors, which may contribute to the final pregnancy outcome. Factors that should be taken into consideration include the age of the woman, the obstetric history, the size and position of the fetus, current midwifery and obstetric practice, and the use of analgesia during labour.

## Birth outcome and birthweight

There is concern that physical training may adversely affect the development of the fetus. However, findings from many studies have alleviated this concern to some extent because changes in fetal heart rate noted during maternal exercise were transient and did not interfere with normal fetal growth and development. The well-being of the fetus was considered during this present study, although the physiological effects of pregnancy were not investigated during this study.

Research findings are inconsistent in relation to the Apgar scores of babies at birth and to birthweight. Findings from the current study reported no significant difference between the two groups of participants in terms of Apgar score of the baby at 1 and 5 minutes after birth and of birthweight.

The Apgar score is a routine initial assessment made after delivery, which gives an immediate indication of the general condition of the newborn. These findings agree with the findings of the available literature that there is no significant difference in the Apgar score of babies and birthweight between women who exercised during pregnancy and women in a control group (Collings et al. 1983; Kupla et al. 1987; Botkin and Driscoll 1991; Rose et al. 1991; Lee 1996; Sternfield 1997; Kardel and Kase 1998). It was positive for the researcher to find no reports in the literature of any differences in Apgar scores of babies among sedentary participants, exercising participants and control participants.

Findings in the current literature are controversial in relation to birthweight and maternal physical activity. Current evidence appears to indicate that participation in moderate-to-vigorous activity throughout pregnancy may enhance birthweight, whereas more severe regimes may result in lighter infants. This can give cause for concern in terms of the mortality and morbidity of smaller for gestational age in the event of pre-term delivery.

Findings from the present study indicated that there was no significant difference in birthweight of babies born to participants in both the intervention group and the control group. The range of birthweight was comparable between the two groups with none of the babies, born to participants who completed the study, being born small enough to be classified as low birthweight, i.e. < 2.5 kg. These findings agree with similar findings in birthweight from numerous other studies over the past 20 years.

In contrast to the present findings, other investigators have reported that babies born to exercising mothers were significantly lower in weight than babies born to non-exercising mothers (Bell et al. 1995; Clapp et al. 1998b). Other findings suggest that babies born to mothers who are moderately trained have significantly heavier babies than non-trained or highly trained mothers (Hatch et al. 1993; Bell et al. 1995).

The previous studies discussed were undertaken using differing research designs. This present study included only healthy first-time prospective mothers who continued to be healthy during pregnancy. These are important factors to consider when comparing these findings on birthweight with findings from other studies.

There is the possibility that the well-being of small babies may be compromised. This becomes more of a concern to health professionals and mothers for those babies with a birthweight < 2.5 kg. However, women may associate a smaller baby with an easier labour and think of this as a desirable prospect. In light of this fact, more conclusive evidence is needed to provide further information for women and to assist health professionals to give appropriate advice related to exercise during pregnancy. In addition, more evidence is also needed to support research findings in relation to the effects of exercise on maternal and neonatal anthropometry. It is important to make comparisons of findings with a similar group, and care should be taken to avoid the inappropriate generalisation of research findings.

Limitations in the current literature include the lack of follow-up investigations of those participants who failed to complete exercise studies, and to what extent participants in the control group took part in regular physical activity. The current study attempted to address these limitations. Pregnancy and birth outcomes of those participants who failed to complete the study were investigated. No significant differences were noted in terms of pregnancy and birth outcomes, which included length of gestation, duration of labour, mode of delivery, maternal and baby complications, Apgar score and birth-weight.

Findings of the present study support the findings of other researchers. Healthy pregnant participants may take part in exercise during pregnancy without compromising fetal growth and develop-ment, as judged by Apgar score, birthweight, or complications during the course of pregnancy and labour.

In summary, this present study was undertaken with healthy prospective first-time mothers who were recruited into the study with conservative medical and obstetric inclusion criteria. None of the participants was deemed 'at risk' for obstetric and medical complica-tions, and health and welfare were closely monitored for the duration of the study. In this respect, it was not anticipated that they were likely to develop any complications during pregnancy. These factors may have contributed to the positive outcomes experienced with all pregnancy and birth outcomes.

It can be concluded from the findings of the present study and previous studies that regular moderate exercise during pregnancy undertaken by healthy women remains safe for mother and baby, with women having the benefit of maintaining psychological well-being. Pregnancy should be regarded as a normal event for healthy women and not as a state of confinement. In the absence of medical conditions or obstetric complications, women should be encouraged to continue an active lifestyle during pregnancy.

## Physical activity and retention of participants

In this present study, participants in the control group continued with the existing antenatal preparation for pregnancy, childbirth and the transition to parenthood. Participants in the intervention group additionally took part in a structured exercise programme during and after pregnancy. The study did not prevent participants in either group from continuing with their normal levels of physical activity. Episodes of physical activity undertaken by the participants in the control group and additional episodes of exercise undertaken by the participants in the intervention group were recorded in activity diaries during the study.

No significant difference was noted between the two groups in early pregnancy in relation to how participants described their activity levels. On completion of the study, a significant difference was found between the two groups in relation to the total number of episodes of physical activity undertaken from early pregnancy until 4 months after delivery. The participants in the intervention group were noted to have taken part in significantly more episodes of physical activity than the control participants. This significant difference was noted in the number of sessions of activity that were undertaken, in addition to the structured exercise programme. Both groups of participants tended to report taking part in similar types of activity.

No relationship was found between the frequency of physical activity undertaken during the study and the response of three psychological indicators assessing the perceptions of positive psychological well-being, negative psychological well-being and physical well-being.

Several possible factors contributed to the increased frequency of episodes of physical activity reported by the participants in the intervention group. The regular weekly contact with the exercise instructor and attendance at the structured exercise class may have influenced individual participants to adopt a more active lifestyle. This may incorporate stimulation of the participants to take part in other forms of physical activity. Other factors include: the benefits experienced by participation in the activity itself; the social interaction with other pregnant women; the motivation from group interaction; the relationship with the class instructor; and being in a research study or the habitual nature of the twice-weekly classes.

Participants in the control group also continued to take part in physical activities, but this was significantly reduced when compared with the participants in the intervention group. Associated factors may include the lack of motivation or encouragement from peers, reluctance to attend activities, lack of opportunity to attend relevant activities or limited contact with the researcher.

No significant relationship was found between the frequency of activity sessions and the responses in selected psychological indicators of well-being after pregnancy. This suggests that some factors other than frequency of physical activity may influence psychological well-being of individuals. This may encompass the quality, type and format of exercise programmes undertaken by participants.

The retention of participants within the present study was always a concern, especially when considering the nature and duration (52 weeks) of the study. No statistical difference was found between the two groups in relation to the drop-out rate of participants during the study (i.e. 36% for participants in the control group and 39% for participants in the intervention group). Most of the participants in both groups who dropped out of the study did so in early pregnancy immediately after recruitment (i.e. 29% from the control group and 33% from the intervention group). It is common for randomized controlled trials to lose participants, especially if they are allocated to a group that the participant finds undesirable (Ward and Morgan 1984). This factor may have contributed to this immediate drop-out of participants from both groups, with those wishing to exercise being recruited to the control group and those not wishing to exercise being allocated to the intervention group.

The drop-out rate of participants from randomized controlled trials has been estimated to be 20% and possibly as high as 40% (Ward and Morgan 1984). The drop-out rate from the present study, although high, was within the accepted range for randomized controlled trials. Steptoe (1992) identifies the maximum retention of participants in exercise studies as 80–85%, even in populations with good facilities and with participants who have positive attitudes towards exercise. He suggests that the crucial problem for randomized controlled trials of psychological response is not so much that the drop-out rate should be minimized, but that the drop-out rate should not be selective across experimental conditions (Steptoe 1992).

In summary, the women in the intervention group participated in a higher number of exercise sessions during the study compared with the control participants. There was no significant relationship found between the frequency of activity sessions and the responses in selected psychological indicators after pregnancy. Factors that may have influenced participants to remain in the study and undertake further activity included: the psychological and physical benefits gained from the exercise programme itself, the group interaction and social interaction with other pregnant women, participation in a research study, and the enthusiasm, positive reinforcement and motivation gained from the exercise instructor and other pregnant participants.

# Summary of the discussion

Women are expected to experience a reduction in psychological well-being during pregnancy. This is regarded as typical and a normal feature of pregnancy, and it does not imply any poor psychological adjustment. Findings from this present study suggest that women who participate in regular physical activity during pregnancy experience a maintenance or delay in reduction of levels of psychological well-being during pregnancy. This is in contrast to the significant deterioration in psychological well-being experienced by participants in the control group during the same period.

No differences were found between the participants in both groups in relation to pregnancy and birth outcomes. Findings for pregnancy and birth outcomes were similar for those participants who did not complete the study. Participants in both groups experienced positive pregnancy and birth outcomes. There were no major maternal or neonatal complications reported during pregnancy and childbirth. One subject from the intervention group experienced a complication six weeks postpartum that was directly related to the type of delivery.

The women in the intervention group participated in a significantly higher number of exercise sessions during the study. No significant relationship was found between the frequency of activity sessions and the responses in selected psychological indicators after pregnancy. This finding suggests that factors other than the frequency of physical activity sessions influenced these findings.

The psychological benefit gained by the participants in the intervention group might have been influenced directly by the exercise itself or indirectly by other factors. Possible influencing factors include psychosocial support, group interaction and participation in a research study.

Most published studies discussed within this section have suffered from limitations in the research design. In particular, participant selection bias and lack of control participants limited the application of findings only to active women. These study design problems made it difficult to compare both the findings from the present study and the results from different studies. Both the present study and other research studies discussed have contributed significantly to current knowledge and understanding of the effects of exercise on pregnancy, and have raised issues for further investigation.

The findings of the present study offer support to the findings from research studies of exercise during pregnancy. Women who exercise regularly during pregnancy will experience positive psychological wellbeing. Healthy women may exercise safely during pregnancy without any additional risk to the woman, pregnancy or baby.

# Chapter 6
# Conclusions

This chapter provides a brief summary of the current situation in relation to women who wish to exercise during pregnancy. The need for further research is highlighted in order to develop further knowledge and understanding of the impact of exercise on pregnancy. A summary of the main conclusions to the present study is presented, along with implications for practice and areas identified for further research.

There is general agreement that regular exercise has physical, psychological and health benefits, which can enhance the quality of life for individuals. Considering these benefits, it is understandable that women of child-bearing years now wish to continue with or adopt an active lifestyle during pregnancy. The benefits gained from regular exercise may help women to prepare both mentally and physically for the emotional and physical challenges inherent in pregnancy and childbirth.

Pregnancy is a unique state and involves profound physiological and psychological changes, which can create special risks that do not affect non-pregnant women. This raises important fundamental questions for the women themselves, health professionals and exercise scientists. These questions include the ways in which pregnancy alters a woman's ability to exercise, how much exercise is safe, and to what extent exercise influences the course and outcome of pregnancy and the development of the fetus.

Recent national strategies promote regular activity to the general population as a means of maintaining and improving health. In particular, women are identified as a target group as a result of the specific benefits to women's health. In light of these developments, there is need to investigate further the effects of exercise during pregnancy through scientific research. If healthy active lifestyles are to be encouraged, health professionals involved in developing maternity strategies need to consider these within antenatal education programmes. Women should be supported if they wish to adopt active lifestyles during pregnancy and appropriate opportunities should be made available to allow them to exercise safely.

The present study was undertaken to address some of these important issues. Findings have highlighted that those women who exercised regularly during pregnancy experienced benefits in psychological well-being compared with women in the control group. There were no differences noted between the groups in relation to pregnancy and birth outcomes.

## Conclusions of the study

The results of the study have been established in relation to the comparison of healthy prospective first-time mothers who continued with the existing antenatal education programme with women who also participated in regular physical activity from early pregnancy until four months after delivery of the baby.

Regular physical activity during pregnancy and after pregnancy has benefits to the psychological well-being of women by maintaining early pregnancy levels of psychological well-being in terms of perceptions of coping assets (positive psychological well-being) and coping deficits (negative psychological well-being), physical well-being, somatic symptoms experienced and body image.

Regular physical activity during and after pregnancy has benefits to psychological well-being of women by maintaining or delaying a reduction in early pregnancy levels of psychological well-being in terms of attitudes to marital relationships, attitudes to sex, and attitudes to the pregnancy and the baby.

Regular physical activity during pregnancy does not significantly influence postnatal emotional well-being/depression, although exercise is associated with more positive emotional well-being. There was no significant relationship between the total amount of physical activity and the responses to the psychological indicators of well-being after pregnancy.

Regular physical activity during pregnancy does not influence pregnancy or birth outcomes in terms of the length of gestation, duration of labour and mode of delivery, birthweight and neonatal well-being, as assessed by the Apgar score at birth. Regular physical activity during pregnancy does not influence maternal or neonatal complications.

Therefore, it can be concluded from the findings of the current study that regular exercise has positive psychological advantages for pregnant women and there are no risks in terms of health of the fetus or birth outcome.

# Recommendations for practice

The following recommendations for practice are made in light of current knowledge of the effects of exercise and pregnancy and on the results of the present study.

Health professionals and exercise instructors should have access to current and up-to-date information about the effects of exercise on pregnancy. This would enable them to provide accurate information and advice to meet the individual needs of pregnant woman. Knowledge in this area would provide an opportunity to promote an active lifestyle.

In-service training should be provided to raise awareness of the physical and psychological benefits to be gained by women from participation in regular exercise. Information should be widely available on current guidelines and local practices in relation to exercise during pregnancy and the provision of services available locally.

Midwives, in particular, should incorporate the effects of exercise and pregnancy within their continued personal professional development. This would ensure that their knowledge and understanding were updated and their practice was based on current research findings. This would enable them confidently to provide appropriate information and advice to pregnant women attending for midwifery care.

Providers of maternity services should ensure that exercise opportunities are incorporated within the existing antenatal education programmes. There should be close liaison with local leisure centres or other providers of exercise to be aware of, or involved with, the provisions available.

Appropriate training in antenatal and postnatal exercise for midwife practitioners involved with pregnant women should be available to allow those midwives with a special interest in this area to become fully qualified instructors.

Exercise instructors and health advisors who may be involved with women who exercise during pregnancy should have access to regular training updates. This is required to enable them to appropriately advise and provide safe and effective exercise.

# Further research

Over research decades, a wealth of literature has emerged which investigates the effects of exercise on fetal and maternal well-being during pregnancy and birth outcome. The present study has shown that healthy women who exercise regularly during pregnancy experience maintenance of psychological well-being, with no risk to either pregnancy or the baby. However, further research is needed in this area to enable conclusions to be drawn and to provide further knowledge and understanding of the impact of exercise on pregnancy.

It would be an advantage to have further information available to allow the parameters of safe and appropriate exercise levels to be defined. These parameters should consider all categories of pregnant women in terms of exercise history, present health and activity levels, and obstetric and medical history.

It would be of interest to investigate the extent to which pregnant women adhere to exercise programmes. This should include reasons why women do or do not continue with an exercise programme. This information would contribute to knowledge and understanding of adherence to exercise programmes during pregnancy and would allow the necessary intervention to the provision of programmes.

More conclusive information is required to detect potential effects on maternal and infant health. The effects of exercise on fetal growth, gestational age and duration of labour are of particular importance. Studies in this area would need to be well controlled to provide conclusive information that can be generalized to other pregnant women.

Information is needed to provide information about psychological well-being in both the antenatal and postnatal periods. Current research suggests that exercise provides psychological benefits and this would be an advantage to women during this important life event. A further area of interest would be during the intranatal period. Research should investigate whether exercise influences women in relation to coping strategies during labour, subjective experience of labour and perceptions of pain.

Research findings suggest that exercise promotes mental health and prevents depression. Therefore, research should be extended to investigate further the effects of exercise on the mental health of women during pregnancy and the role exercise may have in the prevention of postnatal depression.

Future studies need to be well controlled to enable research findings to be generalized to pregnant women. Therefore, consideration should be given to address the recognized limitations evident in current literature, i.e. appropriate sample size, history, type and intensity of exercise during pregnancy, consideration of incidence of complications, change in weight, body composition and appropriate statistical calculations undertaken to allow application of the data to the general population.

## Final note from the researcher

It is now over a decade since I first started to plan this research study. At the time, there was little provision for women to exercise during pregnancy, and health professionals and maternity service providers did not see this as an issue of concern. I remained firm in my belief that everyone who wanted to have an active lifestyle should experience the benefits of exercise, including women during pregnancy.

In the face of adversity, I proceeded with my venture with the help of a few supporters. The study was planned, piloted, commenced and completed. Over this time, the study caught the interest and attention of a variety of individuals. An increasing number of women, midwives, obstetricians, physiotherapists and exercise instructors began to seek further information. On the whole, all interest about exercise and pregnancy was of a positive nature.

I am now delighted to say that many changes have taken place locally in a short period of time. Attitudes towards women who want to remain active are more positive. Women are supported and given more appropriate information. There are more opportunities for women to exercise during pregnancy. Provisions are available in the local health and fitness centres, and some midwives have trained as exercise instructors and now provide classes. More and more, individuals are contacting me for advice and guidance about exercise-related issues. This includes women and health professionals such as midwives and general practitioners. The variety of issues includes clarification about what would be the most appropriate type and amount of exercise for individual women, contraindications and information about the provision of exercise for pregnancy.

The present study, together with my earlier work in this field of interest, is my contribution to the promotion of a healthy lifestyle. This is only the start, because the work must continue. More research is needed to ensure that findings are more conclusive. It has been a privilege and a pleasure to be involved in this study. I welcome contact from anyone who is interested in this field.

# Appendices

## Appendix 1: participant recruitment letter

Dear [Mother to Be]

I am undertaking a research study in conjunction with Ayrshire Central Hospital and the University of Glasgow. The information obtained from this study may have a valuable contribution when planning future developments in antenatal care.

The study may only require women to undertake the existing available antenatal care offered to pregnant women or **in addition** to this care some women may be asked to undertake a regular exercise programme. The exercise class, taken by myself, will be held within Ayrshire Central Hospital. All women in the study will be asked to complete a **total** of three questionnaires during and following pregnancy.

Please indicate below if you are interested in taking part in this study. This will be discussed with your consultant obstetrician at the appointment today. Your obstetrician will decide whether you are fit, healthy and suitable to participate in the study.

If agreed, then you will be given a sealed envelope containing further information of your group in the study. The first questionnaire will be enclosed for you to complete and return.

Thank you for taking the time to read this letter,

Yours sincerely

*Jean Rankin*

*Tear Off* —————————————————————————————————

**Please circle your response below and return this slip to the Reception desk.**
*I am interested or* **I am NOT interested**          *in taking part in this study*

*NAME* _____          *DATE* _____

# Appendix 2: consent form to consultant obstetrician

**Re:** _____

*Dear Doctor* _____

The above woman has consented to take part in the research study that aims to investigate the *'Effects of Exercise during Pregnancy'*.

The woman will be randomly assigned to one of the following two groups:

The **'control'** group of participants will continue with the existing antenatal preparation for childbirth and motherhood.

**OR**

The **'intervention'** group of participants will undertake a structured and supervised exercise class at ACH **in addition to** the existing antenatal preparation for childbirth and motherhood.

I would be obliged if you would agree to her participation in the study.

Yours sincerely,

*Jean Rankin*

I **consent/do not consent** to this woman participating in this study.

Signature of Consultant _____Date _____

**Please retain this form in the medical notes**

# Appendix 3: information letter to general practitioner/midwife

**re:** _____

Dear Doctor/Sister_____

The above woman has consented to take part in a research study at Ayrshire Central Hospital, Irvine, which has received ethical approval from Ayrshire and Arran Health Board. Consent for participation in the study has also been obtained from her consultant obstetrician.

The study is carried out in conjunction with the University of Glasgow and aims to investigate the *Effects of Exercise during Pregnancy.*

The woman has been assigned to:

1. The **'control'** group of participants who have the existing antenatal preparation for childbirth and motherhood.

**OR**

2. The **'intervention'** group of participants who will undertake structured and supervised exercise class at Ayrshire Central Hospital **in addition** to the existing antenatal preparation for childbirth and motherhood.

Please do not hesitate to contact me if you wish to discuss this study further.

Yours sincerely,

*Jean Rankin*
*Senior Midwife*

# Appendix 4: consent form to participants in the control group

I consent to take part in this study and confirm that I have been given the following information:

- My obstetrician has agreed that I am fit and healthy and can participate in the study.
- My general practitioner and named midwife can be informed with my permission.
- It has been explained to me that I will be offered all available existing antenatal care during my pregnancy.
- I am aware that I will be asked to complete a total of three questionnaires during and following pregnancy and I have received information giving me further details.
- I am aware that details of any complications, hospital admissions, labour and birth outcomes may be obtained from my medical notes for use in the study.
- I have been given a telephone number to contact if I have any questions.
- I am aware that I can discontinue with this study at any stage.
- I understand that all information will be confidential.

*Signature of Subject* _____*Date*_____

*Signature of Researcher* _____*Date*_____

**Copy to: Subject/Researcher/Medical notes**

# Appendix 5: consent form to participants in the intervention group

I consent to take part in this study and confirm that I have been given the following information:

- My obstetrician has agreed that I am fit and healthy and can participate in the study.
- My general practitioner and named midwife may be informed with my permission.
- It has been explained to me that I will undertake a structured exercise programme during and following pregnancy and I have received an information leaflet that gives me further details of the exercise programme.
- I am aware that I can discontinue with the exercise class if I have any concerns and I will also be advised to stop the exercise programme immediately if I develop any complications during pregnancy.
- I am aware that I will be asked to complete a total of three questionnaires during and following pregnancy and I have received information giving me further details.
- I am aware that details of any complications, hospital admissions, labour and birth outcomes may be obtained from my medical notes for use in the study.
- I have been given a telephone number to contact if I have any questions.
- I am aware that I can discontinue with this study at anytime.
- I understand that all information will be confidential.

*Signature of Participant* _____*Date*_____

*Signature of Researcher* _____*Date*_____

**Copy to: Participant/Researcher/Medical notes**

# Appendix 6: information letter to participants in the control group

*Thank you for agreeing to participate in the study.*

- You have been assigned to the **'control'** group of participants who will continue with the **existing available antenatal care** during pregnancy.
- Your consultant obstetrician has agreed to your participation in this study because you are a healthy women with a healthy pregnancy.
- Your midwifery and medical notes will have an identification sticker attached to let midwifery/medical staff know that you are in this study.
- I will monitor the progress of your pregnancy by keeping in contact with either yourself, consultant obstetrician or your medical notes.
- I may need to collect information from your medical notes about any hospital admissions or any complications you may have during pregnancy.
- Details of your pregnancy, delivery and birth may also be obtained from your medical notes for use in the study.
- You will be asked to complete a booklet of questions asking you how you are feeling about yourself and your pregnancy on **three** separate occasions during and following pregnancy.
- Your first questionnaire is in the information envelope and the next two questionnaires will be sent to your home address by post. A stamped addressed envelope with my address will also be issued to allow you to return the completed questionnaire to me.
- Please keep your activity diary up to date. You should include the following information that will be helpful to you when you summarize your physical activities on the three questionnaires: Type of physical activity, duration and frequency of the activity. A total of all exercise classes attended. Do not hesitate to contact me if you need to discuss any forms of physical activities you have undertaken or wish to undertake.

- All information about you will be kept confidential.
- All information recorded under a personal code number (on the front of your envelope).
- You are able to leave the study at any time you wish.
- Please contact me at the telephone number above if you wish to discuss the study further.

*Thank you for your co-operation.*

*Jean Rankin*

# Appendix 7: information letter to participants in the intervention group

*Thank you for agreeing to participate in this study.*

- You have been assigned to the **intervention group** of participants.
- Your consultant obstetrician has agreed to your participation in this study because you are a healthy women with a healthy pregnancy.
- This means that you will have the existing available antenatal care offered to women during your pregnancy and **in addition** you will be asked to undertake **a structured exercise programme** during and following pregnancy.
- The exercise programme used in the class is especially designed for pregnant women. Exercises will consist of gentle warm up, moderate aerobic exercises, stretching and body conditioning, and cool down. The session lasts for between 40 and 45 minutes. You may wear any comfortable clothes *e.g. tee shirt and leggings*.
- The exercise class will be held twice weekly in Ayrshire Central Hospital. **In addition** you may undertake other physical activities *e.g.* aquanatal which is offered weekly at your local leisure centre, brisk walking or cycling. Videotapes of an exercise programme specifically designed for pregnancy and following birth are available for home use. Do not hesitate to contact me if you need to discuss any forms of physical activities you have undertaken or wish to undertake.
- It is advised that exercise should be undertaken **three times per week.** It is advised that the exercise session should be attended whenever possible, preferably twice per week or at least once per week.
- You may discontinue with the exercise classes at any time if you have any concerns and you will be asked to discontinue with the exercise programme immediately if you have developed any complications during your pregnancy.
- Your midwifery and medical notes will have an identification sticker attached to let midwifery/medical staff know that you are participating in this study.
- I will monitor the progress of your pregnancy by keeping in contact with either yourself, consultant obstetrician or from your medical notes.
- Details of your pregnancy, delivery and birth may also be obtained from your medical notes for use in the study.
- I may need to collect information from your medical notes about any hospital admissions or any complications you may have during pregnancy.
- You will be asked to complete a booklet of questions asking you how you are feeling about yourself and your pregnancy on **three** separate occasions during and following pregnancy.
- Your first questionnaire is in the information envelope and the next two questionnaires will be sent to your home address by post. A stamped addressed envelope with my address will also be issued to allow you to return the completed questionnaire to me.
- Please keep your activity diary up to date. You should include the following information that will be helpful to you when you summarize your physical

activities on the three questionnaires: Type of physical activity, duration and frequency of the activity. A register is maintained of your attendance at the hospital classes.

- All information about you will be kept confidential.
- All information recorded under a personal code number (on the front of your envelope).
- You are able to leave the study at any time you wish.

Please contact me at the telephone number above if you wish to discuss the study further.

*Thank you for your cooperation.*

*Jean Rankin*

# Appendix 8: information letter about questionnaires

*Dear_____,*

*Thank you for taking the time to participate in this study.*

*I have enclosed questionnaire number _____ for you to complete and return in the SAE provided.*

**Just a reminder about the study:**
The study is voluntary and you are under no obligation to continue.
This study is designed for first time mothers only.

Information will be obtained to find out about your physical well-being and how you are feeling about yourself, your pregnancy, your body and your relationships.

During the study you will complete a total of three of these questionnaires:

1. In early pregnancy when you join the study
2. During the last few weeks of pregnancy
3. Finally 12–16 weeks after your baby is born

In addition you are asked to keep an activity diary or record of your physical activity on a weekly/monthly basis and give brief details of your labour/delivery.

**About the questionnaire:**
It will take about 10–15 minutes to complete.

Please answer the questions promptly.

You will be asked to write a brief summary of your physical activity from your personal diary. All exercise classes attended will be totalled at the end of the study.

*Please contact me if you wish to discuss any aspects of the study, if you do not wish to continue with the study or to keep me up to date with your activities or let me know when your baby is born.*

*If I do not hear from you then I will send out your next questionnaire routinely.*

*I hope you are keeping well,*

**Jean Rankin**

# Appendix 9: interpretation of questions

**Interpretation of questions: this page section is for data analysis only**

Scoring of the Outcome Variables in the Questionnaire
*Perceptions of coping assets (positive psychological well-being)*
14 questions in total. Range of individual scores = 0 – 4.

Total score = 56 (higher score is positive)

Questions 1, 3, 5, 10, 11, 13, 15, 16, 18, 19, 20, 22, 23, 29

*Perceptions of coping deficits (negative psychological well-being)*
10 questions in total. Range of individual scores = 0 – 4.

Questions 2, 4, 6, 8, 9, 12, 14, 17, 21, 28

Total score = 40 (higher score is negative)

**Rotate question 6**

*Perceptions of physical well-being*
6 questions in total. Range of individual scores = 0 – 4. Total score = 24
(higher score is positive). Questions 7, 24, 25, 26, 27, 30

**MAMA subscales** Scores 1 – 2 = undesirable responses. Scores 3 – 4 = desirable responses (for the purpose of this study **only** the direction of the positive and negative scores were rotated from the original author)

*Perceptions of body image*
Questions 2, 12, 18, 19, 21, 31, 44, 47, 49, 53, 55, 57

**Rotate questions 2, 12, 19, 21, 49, 53, 55 and 57**

*Perceptions of somatic symptoms*
Questions 1, 4, 6, 9, 17, 27, 32, 33, 35, 38, 41, 59

**Rotate questions 1, 17, 33 and 41**

*Attitudes to marital relationships*
Questions 3, 8, 15, 26, 34, 36, 37, 43, 48, 50, 52, 56

**Rotate questions 8, 34, 36, 37, 48 and 56**

*Attitudes to sex*
Questions 5, 11, 13, 20, 23, 25, 30, 39, 42, 45, 46, 58

**Rotate questions 5, 13, 20, 23, 42, 45 and 58**

*Attitudes to pregnancy/baby*
Questions 7, 10, 14, 16, 22, 24, 28, 29, 40, 51, 54, 60

**Rotate questions 24, 28, 29, 40 and 60**

*Edinburgh Postnatal Depression Scale*
Scores 1–10. Lower score is the more positive response. Score of individual questions = 0–3. Total score = 30

## Appendix 10: questionnaire booklet

## Code No: _____

MAMA

# QUESTIONNAIRE

Name: _____        Date: _____

Group: _____        Questionnaire No: _____

No. of weeks of pregnancy: _____        EDD: _____

*No of weeks since delivery:*        *Date of Delivery:* _____

- *Thank you for taking the time to complete this questionnaire.*
- *Please use the back cover for any comments or messages.*
- *All information will be treated in confidence.*
- *Please return to Jean Rankin in the envelope provided.*

### Summary of Physical Activity

*Review your activities over the past four weeks from your activity diary.*

1. Would you please **circle** the response which you feel best describes your present level of physical activity, *e.g. aquanatal; swimming; exercise classes; cycling, gym work, sports, hobbies, etc.*
- *Inactive,* i.e. *You have not taken any form of physical activity at all.*
- *Occasionally active,* i.e. *You have taken physical activity on an occasion only and not on any regular basis.*
- *Regularly active,* i.e. *You have regular set episodes of activity or exercise, daily or weekly, etc.*
- *Very active,* i.e. *You are exercising almost every day or every other day.*

*Summary of Physical Activity Exercise Diary*
2. Would you please **circle** the response that best describes the average times you have taken any form of physical activity per week:

*None        once        twice        three times        more than three times*

3. List the types of physical activity you have undertaken:
*On a regular basis:        How often        Occasionally        How often*
*in one month:        taken?        in one month:*

4. Please **circle** the statement that describes your intention to alter your level of physical activity:

I intend to increase        I intend to decrease        I intend to keep the
                                                        same level of activity

5.  Please **circle** the statement that describes how you have been during or following
    pregnancy:
    **Yes**, I have kept well        **No**, I have not kept well
    Reason, if unwell:

6.  Please give **brief details** of any hospital stays:

| Length of stay: | Weeks of pregnancy/ postnatal | Reason |
|---|---|---|
|  |  |  |

**Remember to keep a record of all your activity especially any classes you
have attended. These details will be required at the end of the study.**

## Well-being

Below is a list of words and phrases that describe feelings that people have. Please read
**each one carefully**, then circle the response that best describes the extent to which
you have had this feeling **during the past week including today.**

During the last week and including today **to what extent have you been feeling:**

1.  Self confident   Not at all   A little   Moderately   Quite a lot   Extremely
2.  Easily irritated  Not at all   A little   Moderately   Quite a lot   Extremely
3.  Enthusiastic    Not at all   A little   Moderately   Quite a lot   Extremely
4.  Disappointed    Not at all   A little   Moderately   Quite a lot   Extremely
    with yourself
5.  Uplifted        Not at all   A little   Moderately   Quite a lot   Extremely
6.  Calm            Not at all   A little   Moderately   Quite a lot   Extremely
7.  Refreshed       Not at all   A little   Moderately   Quite a lot   Extremely
8.  Drained         Not at all   A little   Moderately   Quite a lot   Extremely
9.  Easily upset    Not at all   A little   Moderately   Quite a lot   Extremely
10. Proud of        Not at all   A little   Moderately   Quite a lot   Extremely
    yourself
11. Elated          Not at all   A little   Moderately   Quite a lot   Extremely
12. Distressed      Not at all   A little   Moderately   Quite a lot   Extremely
13. Invigorated     Not at all   A little   Moderately   Quite a lot   Extremely
14. Bothered        Not at all   A little   Moderately   Quite a lot   Extremely

**To what extent have you been feeling that you are:**

15. Coping          Not at all   A little   Moderately   Quite a lot   Extremely
16. Achieving       Not at all   A little   Moderately   Quite a lot   Extremely
    something
17. Overwhelmed  Not at all   A little   Moderately   Quite a lot   Extremely

| 18. Overcoming difficulties | Not at all | A little | Moderately | Quite a lot | Extremely |
|---|---|---|---|---|---|
| 19. Getting closer to your goals | Not at all | A little | Moderately | Quite a lot | Extremely |
| 20. Well organized | Not at all | A little | Moderately | Quite a lot | Extremely |
| 21. Under too much pressure | Not at all | A little | Moderately | Quite a lot | Extremely |
| 22. Competent | Not at all | A little | Moderately | Quite a lot | Extremely |
| 23. Getting things under control | Not at all | A little | Moderately | Quite a lot | Extremely |

**To what extent have you been feeling physically:**

| 24. Healthy | Not at all | A little | Moderately | Quite a lot | Extremely |
|---|---|---|---|---|---|
| 25. Strong | Not at all | A little | Moderately | Quite a lot | Extremely |
| 26. Supple | Not at all | A little | Moderately | Quite a lot | Extremely |
| 27. Fit | Not at all | A little | Moderately | Quite a lot | Extremely |
| 28. Run down | Not at all | A little | Moderately | Quite a lot | Extremely |
| 29. Attractive | Not at all | A little | Moderately | Quite a lot | Extremely |
| 30. Well | Not at all | A little | Moderately | Quite a lot | Extremely |

## MAMA

*Please complete each question below by putting a circle around the answer that most closely applies to you. Quickly answer each question on how you have been feeling during the past month. If you have not considered some of these questions during the past month then please answer them on your present feelings.*

### IN THE PAST MONTH

1. Have you felt out of breath easily?
   **Very often**        **Often**              **Rarely**           **Never**
2. Have you felt attractive?
   **Never**             **Rarely**             **Often**            **Very often**
3. Has there been a lot of tension between you and your partner, *i.e. irritability, unpleasantness, silence, etc.?*
   **Never**             **Rarely**             **Often**            **Very often**
4. Have you been perspiring a lot?
   **Never**             **Rarely**             **Often**            **Very often**
5. Have you found your partner sexually desirable?
   **Never**             **Rarely**             **Often**            **Very often**
6. Have you vomited?
   **Never**             **Rarely**             **Often**            **Very often**
7. Have you been worrying that you may not be a good mother?
   **Not at all**        **A little**           **A lot**            **Very much**
8. Have arguments between you and your partner come close to blows?
   **Very often**        **Often**              **Rarely**           **Never**
9. Have you felt faint or dizzy?
   **Never**             **Rarely**             **Often**            **Very often**

10. Have you been worrying about hurting your baby inside you?
    **Not at all**  **A little**  **A lot**  **Very much**
11. Do you think your partner has found you sexually desirable?
    **Very often**  **Often**  **Rarely**  **Never**
12. Have you felt that your body smelt nice?
    **Never**  **Rarely**  **Often**  **Very often**
13. Have you looked forward to having sexual intercourse?
    **Not at all**  **A little**  **A lot**  **Very much**
14. Has it worried you that you may not have any time to yourself once your baby is born?
    **Not at all**  **A little**  **A lot**  **Very much**
15. Have you found it easy to show affection to your partner?
    **Very often**  **Often**  **Rarely**  **Never**
16. Have you regretted being pregnant?
    **Never**  **Rarely**  **Often**  **Very often**
17. Have you experienced tingling sensations in your breasts?
    **Very often**  **Often**  **Rarely**  **Never**
18. Have you felt that your breasts were too small?
    **Not at all**  **A little**  **A lot**  **Very much**
19. Have you liked the shape of your body?
    **Not at all**  **A little**  **A lot**  **Very much**
20. Have you felt shy about sex?
    **Very much**  **A lot**  **A little**  **Not at all**
21. Have you felt that your face was attractive?
    **Not at all**  **A little**  **A lot**  **Very much**
22. Has the thought of wearing maternity clothes appealed to you?
    **Very much**  **A lot**  **A little**  **Not at all**
23. Have you felt that having sexual intercourse has been less private because there is a baby inside you?
    **Very much**  **A lot**  **A little**  **Not at all**
24. Have you been feeling happy that you are pregnant?
    **Not at all**  **A little**  **A lot**  **Very much**
25. Have you enjoyed kissing and petting?
    **Very much**  **A lot**  **A little**  **Not at all**
26. Has your partner helped with the running of the house?
    **Very much**  **A lot**  **A little**  **Not at all**
27. Have you suffered from constipation?
    **Never**  **Rarely**  **Often**  **Very often**
28. Has the thought of having more children appealed to you?
    **Not at all**  **A little**  **A lot**  **Very much**
29. Have you felt that pregnancy was unpleasant?
    **Very much**  **A lot**  **A little**  **Not at all**
30. Have you been wondering whether having sexual intercourse might be harmful for baby?
    **Not at all**  **A little**  **A lot**  **Very much**
31. Have you felt that your breasts are too big?
    **Not at all**  **A little**  **A lot**  **Very much**
32. Have you felt full of energy?
    **Very often**  **Often**  **Rarely**  **Never**

33. Have your ankles swollen up?
*Very often*     *Often*     *Rarely*     *Never*

34. Have you felt that your partner was paying you too little attention?
*Very often*     *Often*     *Rarely*     *Never*

35. Have you felt wide-awake in the daytime?
*Very often*     *Often*     *Rarely*     *Never*

36. Has your partner seemed to ignore how you are feeling?
*Very often*     *Often*     *Rarely*     *Never*

37. Has your partner tried to share your interests?
*Never*     *Rarely*     *Often*     *Very often*

38. Have you suffered from indigestion or heartburn?
*Never*     *Rarely*     *Often*     *Very often*

39. Have you felt tense and unhappy at the thought of sexual intercourse?
*Never*     *Rarely*     *Often*     *Very often*

40. Have you been looking forward to caring for your baby's needs?
*Not at all*     *A little*     *A lot*     *Very much*

41. Have you felt nauseated *(felt sick)*?
*Very often*     *Often*     *Rarely*     *Never*

42. Have you felt that sex was unpleasant?
*Very much*     *A lot*     *A little*     *Not at all*

43. Have you felt that your partner went out too often without you?
*Never*     *Rarely*     *Often*     *Very often*

44. Have you felt proud of your appearance?
*Very much*     *A lot*     *A little*     *Not at all*

45. Have you felt that you were easily aroused sexually?
*Never*     *Rarely*     *Often*     *Very often*

46. Have you been having pleasurable daydreams about sex?
*Very often*     *Often*     *Rarely*     *Never*

47. Have you felt that your body was soft and cuddly?
*Very much*     *A lot*     *A little*     *Not at all*

48. Have you been feeling close to your partner since you became pregnant?
*Never*     *Rarely*     *Often*     *Very often*

49. Has your body felt awkward and ungainly?
*Very much*     *A lot*     *A little*     *Not at all*

50. Have you felt like putting your arms around your partner and cuddling him?
*Very much*     *A lot*     *A little*     *Not at all*

51. Have you been wondering whether your baby will be healthy and normal?
*Not at all*     *A little*     *A lot*     *Very much*

52. Has your partner shown affection to you?
*Very often*     *Often*     *Rarely*     *Never*

53. Have you felt that your complexion was poor?
*Very much*     *A lot*     *A little*     *Not at all*

54. Have you felt that life will be difficult after your baby is born?
*Not at all*     *A little*     *A lot*     *Very much*

55. Have you felt that your breasts were attractive?
*Not at all*     *A little*     *A lot*     *Very much*

56. Have you wished that you could rely more on your partner to look after you?
    **Very often**     **Often**          **Rarely**          **Never**
57. Have you felt that you were too fat?
    **Very much**    **A lot**        **A little**        Not at all
58. Have you wanted to have sexual intercourse?
    **Not at all**    **A little**        **A lot**        **Very much**
59. Have you enjoyed your food?
    **Very much**    **A lot**        **A little**        Not at all
60. Has the thought of breast-feeding your baby appealed to you?
    **Not at all**    **A little**        **A lot**        **Very much**

MAMA (postnatal version)
10. Have you been worried about hurting your baby?
14. Have you had enough time for yourself since you had the baby?
16. Have you regretted having the baby?
22. Have you felt proud of being a mother?
23. Have you felt that sexual intercourse is less private now that you have a baby?
24. Have you been feeling happy that you have a baby?
29. Have you felt disappointed by motherhood?
30. Have you felt inhibited about sex since you had the baby?
40. Have you enjoyed caring for your baby's needs?
48. Have you been feeling close to your partner since the baby was born?
54. Has life been more difficult since the baby was born?
60. Have you enjoyed feeding your baby?

## Edinburgh Postnatal Depression Scale

*Underline or circle the* **one** *response to* **each** *of the following questions that comes closest to how you have felt* **over the past seven days** *and* **not just** *how you feel today.*

1. *I have been able to laugh and see the funny side of things:*
   As much as I always could          Definitely not so much now
   Not quite so much now              Not at all

2. *I have looked forward with enjoyment to things:*
   As much as I ever did              Definitely less than I used to
   Rather less than I used to         Hardly at all

3. *I have blamed myself unnecessarily when things go wrong:*
   Yes, most of the time              Not very often
   Yes, some of the time              No, never

4. *I have felt worried and anxious for no good reason:*
   No, not at all                     Hardly ever
   Yes, sometimes                     Yes, always

5. *I have felt scared or panicky for no good reason:*
   Yes, quite a lot                   No, not much
   Yes, sometimes                     No, not at all

6. *Things have been getting on top of me:*
   Yes, most of the time I haven't been able to cope at all
   Yes, sometimes I haven't been coping as well as usual
   No, most of the time I have coped          No, I have been
   quite well                                 coping as well as ever

7. *I have been so unhappy that I have had difficulty sleeping:*
   Yes, most of the time                      Not very often
   Yes, sometimes                             No, not at all

8. *I have felt sad or miserable:*
   Yes, most of the time                      Not very often
   Yes, quite often                           No, not at all

9. *I have been so unhappy that I have been crying:*
   Yes, most of the time                      Only occasionally
   Yes, quite often                           No, never

10. *The thought of harming myself has occurred to me:*
    Yes, quite often                          Hardly ever
    Sometimes                                 Never

**Please give brief details of your labour and delivery**
How many weeks pregnant were you? _____

Did you start labour yourself or were you induced?_____
Duration of labour: _____hours

Details of any pain relief: _____

Type of delivery: *Normal, forceps, arranged section, emergency section, other:*
_____

Did you need any stitches? _____ Why? _____

Did **you** have any problems? _____

Baby's date of birth: _____ Boy/Girl: _____

Birthweight _____

Did you have any problems with baby? _____

How are you feeding baby? _____ How long did you stay in hospital? _____

*Comments, use the back to write additional comments*

## Appendix 11: activity diary

Code number: _____ Date baby is due: _____ Birth date of baby: _____

| Month | Type of Exercise | Duration | How often? |
|---|---|---|---|
| Week 1 | | | |
| Week 2 | | | |
| Week 3 | | | |
| Week 4 | | | |

*This form may be used to record your physical activities.*

# Appendix 12: details of birth outcome

Details of Labour and Birth Outcome
*Subject Code:*

| Labour | | Pain Relief | |
|---|---|---|---|
| POG: _____ | _____weeks | *None: 1 Entonox: 2* | |
| *Spontaneous: 1* | | *Controlled Drug: 3* | |
| *Induced: 2* | _____hours | *Epidural: 4* | |
| *Length:* _____ | | Perineum | |
| Delivery | | *Intact: 1, Tear: 2* | |
| *SVD: 1 Forceps: 2* | | *Episiotomy: 3* | |
| *C/S: Elective: 3* | | | |
| *Emergency: 4* | | | |

**Maternal Complications**

Length of Hospital Stay: _____Days
**Comments:**

| **Sex** | | Birthweight | Apgar Score | Feeding | |
|---|---|---|---|---|---|
| *Girl: 1* | | _____*lb.* _____*oz:* | *1 min.:* ___ | *Breast 1* | |
| *Boy: 2* | | _____*kg* | *5 min:* ____ | *Bottle: 2* | |

**Baby Complications:**

# Appendix 13: exercise class register

*Week beginning:* _____
*Tick where appropriate*

| Code No | Aerobics Mon Fri | | YMCA Video | aqua | swim | brisk walk | Details of any other activities |
|---|---|---|---|---|---|---|---|
| | | | | | | | |
| | | | | | | | |
| | | | | | | | |
| | | | | | | | |
| | | | | | | | |
| | | | | | | | |
| | | | | | | | |
| | | | | | | | |
| | | | | | | | |
| | | | | | | | |
| | | | | | | | |
| | | | | | | | |
| | | | | | | | |
| | | | | | | | |
| | | | | | | | |
| | | | | | | | |
| | | | | | | | |

## Appendix 14: Borg's Category Rating of Perceived Exertion Scale (RPE)

| Rating | Perceived Exertion |
|--------|--------------------|
| 7 | Very Very Light |
| 8 | |
| 9 | Very Light |
| 10 | |
| 11 | Fairly Light |
| 12 | |
| *13 | *Somewhat Hard* |
| *14 | |
| 15 | Hard |
| 16 | |
| 17 | Hard |
| 18 | |
| 19 | Very Very Hard |
| 20 | |

\* Try to exercise within this perceived exertion range.
Do not exercise with a perceived exertion higher than 14.

# References

Alder B (1994) Postnatal Sexuality In: Choi PLY, Nicholson P, eds, *Sexuality: Psychology, Biology and Social Context*. London: Harvester Wheatsheaf.

Allied Dunbar National Fitness Survey (1992) *A summary of major findings of the Allied Dunbar National Fitness Survey*. The Sports Council, Health Education Authority.

American College of Obstetricians and Gynecologists (1994) Exercise during pregnancy and the postpartum period. Technical Bulletin Number 189. *International Federation of Gynecologists Obstetricians* 45 (1): 65–70.

American College of Sports Medicine (1990) The recommended quality and quantity of exercise for developing cardiorespiratory and muscular fitness in adults. *Medicine and Science in Sports and Exercise* 22: 265–74.

Andrews CM, O'Neill LM (1994) Use of pelvic tilt exercise for ligament pain relief *Journal of Nurse Midwife* 39: 370–4.

Araujo D (1997) Expecting questions about exercise and pregnancy? *Physician and Sports Medicine* 25: 85–6, 89–92.

Artal M, Artal Mittlemark R (1991) Emotional aspects of exercise in pregnancy. In: Artal Mittlemark R, Wiswell RA, Drinkwater BL, eds, *Exercise in Pregnancy*. 2nd edn. Baltimore, MD: Willliams & Wilkins, pp. 287–91.

Artal Mittlemark RM, Gardin SK (1991) Historical perspectives In: Artal Mittlemark R, Wiswell RA, Drinkwater BL (1991a) *Exercise in Pregnancy*, 2nd edn. Baltimore, MD: William & Wilkins, pp. 1–7.

Artal R, Sherman C (1999) Exercise during pregnancy: safe and beneficial for most. *Physician and Sports Medicine* 27(8): 51–2, 54, 57–8.

Artal Mittlemark R, Wiswell RA, Drinkwater BL (1991a) *Exercise in Pregnancy*, 2nd edn. Baltimore, MD: Williams & Wilkins.

Artal Mittlemark R, Dorey FJ, Kirschbaum J (1991b) Effects of maternal exercise on pregnancy outcome In: Artal Mittlemark R, Wiswell RA, Drinkwater BL (Eds) *Exercise in Pregnancy*, 2nd edn. Baltimore, MD: William & Wilkins, Chapter 19.

Artal Mittlemark R, Wiswell RA, Drinkwater BL, St Jones-Repovich WE (1991c) Exercise guidelines for pregnancy. In: Artal Mittlemark R, Wiswell RA, Drinkwater BL (Eds) *Exercise in Pregnancy*, 2nd edn. Baltimore, MD: Williams & Wilkins, pp. 299–312.

Ball JA (1989) Postnatal care and adjustments to motherhood. In: *Midwives, Research and Childbirth*, Volume 1. London: Chapman & Hall, pp. 154–75.

178

Barclay ML, McDonald P, O'Loughlan JA (1994) Sexuality and pregnancy: an interview study. *The Australian, New Zealand Journal of Obstetrics and Gynecology* **34**(1): 1–7.

Beck AT, Steer AJ (1979) *Beck Inventory Manual*. New York: Psychological Corporation Jovanovich Inc.

Beckmann CR, Beckmann CA (1990) Effect of a structured antepartum exercise programme on pregnancy and labor outcome in primiparas. *Journal of Reproductive Medicine* **35**: 704–9.

Bell RJ, Palma SM, Lumley JM (1995) The effect of vigorous exercise during pregnancy on birth weight. *Australian, New Zealand Journal of Obstetrics and Gynecology* **35**(1): 46–51.

Bentler PM, Abramson PR (1981) The science of sex research: some methodological considerations. *Archives of Sexual Behaviour* **10**: 225–51.

Berg C, Hammer M, Moller-Nielsen J, Linden W, Thorblad J (1988) Low back pain during pregnancy. *Obstetrics and Gynecology* **71**(1): 71–5.

Berger BG (1984) Running away from anxiety and depression: A female as well as a male race. In: Sachs ML, Buffone GW, eds, *Running as a Therapy*. Lincoln, NB: University of Nebraska Press.

Berlin JA, Colditz GA (1990) Met analysis of physical activity in the prevention of coronary artery disease. *American Journal of Epidemiology* **262**: 2395–401.

Bibring GL (1959) Some considerations of psychological processes in pregnancy and the earliest mother–child relationship. In: *The Psychoanalytic Study of the Child*, volume 14. New York: International University Press, pp. 113–21.

Bibring GL, Dwyer TF, Huntington DS, Valenstein AF (1961) A study of the psychological processes if pregnancy. In: *The Psychoanalytic Study of the Child*, volume 16. New York: International University Press, pp. 9–72.

Blair SN, Kohl HW, Paffenbarger RS, Clark DG, Cooper, KH, Gibbons MD (1989) Physical fitness and all -cause mortality – A prospective study of healthy men and women. *Journal of the American Medical Association* **262**: 2395-2401.

Blankfield A (1967) Is exercise necessary for the obstetric patient? *Medical Journal of Australia* Jan: 163–5.

Botkin C, Driscoll CE (1991) Maternal aerobic exercise: The newborn effects. *Family Practice Research Journal* **11**: 387–93.

Bouchard C, Stephens T (1993) Physical activity, fitness and health: the model and key concepts in physical activity. A consensus statement. In: Bouchard C, Shephard RJ, Stephens T, eds, *Physical Activity, Fitness and Health*. Champaign, IL: Human Kinetics Publishers.

Bouchard C, Shephard RJ, Stephens T (Eds) (1994) *Physical Activity, Fitness and Health*. Champaign, IL: Human Kinetics Publishers.

Brockington IF, Winokur G, Dean C (1982) Puerperal psychosis. In: Brockington IF, Kumar R, eds, *Motherhood and Mental Illness*. London: Academic Press, pp. 37–69.

Brown RD, Harrison JM (1986) The effects of a strength training program on the strength and self concept of two female age groups. *Research Quarterly* **57**: 315–20.

Bung P, Huch R, Huch A (1991) Maternal fetal heart rate patterns in a pregnant athlete during training and laboratory exercise testing: a case report. *European Journal of Obstetrics and Gynecology Reproductive Biology* **39**(1): 59–62.

Burnett C (1956) Value of antenatal exercise. *Journal of Obstetrics and Gynaecology of the British Empire* **63**: 40–57.

Candy M (1994) Raising awareness of a hidden problem: pelvic floor promotion. *Professional Nurse* 9: 280–4.

Capeless EL, Clapp JF (1989) Cardiovascular changes in early pregnancy. *American Journal of Obstetrics and Gynecology* 161: 1449–52.

Carbon R (1994) Female athletes. *British Medical Journal* **309**: 254–8.

Carpenter MW, Sady SP, Hoegsberg B et al. (1988) Fetal heart rate response to maternal exertion. *Journal of American Medical Association* **259**: 3006–9.

Casperson CJ, Powell KE, Christenson GM (1985) Physical activity, exercise and physical fitness: definitions and distinctions for health related research. *Public Health Reports* **100**: 126–31.

Chalmers B (1982) Psychological aspects of pregnancy: Some thoughts for the eighties. *Social Science in Medicine* **16**: 323–31.

Chamberlain G (1991) Work and pregnancy. *British Medical Journal* **302**: 1070.

Cheng D (1996) Preconception health care for the primary care practitioner. *Maryland Medical Journal* **45**: 297–304.

Choi YLP, Mutrie N (1996) The psychological benefits of physical exercise for women: improving employee quality of life. In: Kerr, J, Griffiths A, Cox T, eds, *Workplace Health: Employee fitness and exercise*. London: Taylor & Francis.

Clapp JF (1980) Acute exercise stress in the pregnant ewe. *American Journal of Obstetrics and Gynecology* **136**: 489–94.

Clapp JF (1989) The effects of maternal exercise on early pregnancy outcomes. *American Journal of Obstetrics and Gynecology* **161**: 1453–7.

Clapp JF (1990) The course of labour after endurance exercise during pregnancy. *Obstetrics and Gynecology* **163**: 1799–1805.

Clapp JF (1991a) The changing thermal response to endurance exercise during pregnancy. *American Journal of Obstetrics and Gynecology* **165**: 1684–1689.

Clapp JF (1991b) Maternal exercise performance and early pregnancy outcome. In: Artal Mittlemark R, Wiswell RA, Drinkwater BL, eds, *Exercise in Pregnancy*, 2nd edn. Baltimore, MD: Williams & Wilkins, Chapter 17.

Clapp JF (1994) A clinical approach to exercise during pregnancy. *Clinics in Sports Medicine* **13**: 443–457.

Clapp JF (2000) Exercise during pregnancy: A clinical update. *Clinics in Sports Medicine* **19**: 273–86.

Clapp JF, Capeless EL (1990) Neonatal morphometrics endurance exercise during pregnancy. *American Journal of Obstetrics and Gynecology* **163**: 1805–11.

Clapp JF, Capeless E (1991) The $VO_{2max}$ of recreational athletes before and after pregnancy. *Medicine and Science in Sports and Exercise* **23**: 1128–33.

Clapp JF, Dickstein S (1984) Endurance exercise and pregnancy outcome. *Medicine and Science in Sports and Exercise* **16**: 556–62.

Clapp JF, Rizk KH (1992) Effect of recreational exercise on midtrimester placental growth. *American Journal of Obstetrics and Gynecology* **167**: 1518–23.

Clapp JF, Wesley M, Sleamaker RH (1987) Thermoregulatory and metabolic responses prior to and during pregnancy. *Medicine and Science in Sports and Exercise* **19**: 124–30.

Clapp JF, Little KD, Capeless EL (1993) Fetal heart rate response to sustained recreational exercise. *American Journal of Obstetrics and Gynecology* **168**: 198–206.

Clapp JF, Simonian S, Lopez B, Appleby-Wineberg S, Harcar-Sevcik R (1998a) The one year morphometric and neurodevelopment outcome of the offspring of women who continued to exercise regularly throughout pregnancy. *American Journal of Obstetrics and Gynecology* **178**: 594–9.

Clapp JF, Lopez B, Harcar-Sevcik R (1998b) Neonatal behavioural profile of the offspring of women who continued to exercise regularly throughout pregnancy. *American Journal of Obstetrics and Gynecology* **180**: 91–4.

Clement S, (Ed) (1998) *Psychological Perspectives on Pregnancy and Childbirth.* Edinburgh: Churchill Livingstone.

Cohen GC, Prior JC, Vigna Y, Pride SM (1989) Intense exercise during the first two trimesters of unapparent pregnancy. *Physician Sports Medicine* **17**: 87–91.

Collings CA, Curet LB (1985) Fetal heart rate response to maternal exercise *American Journal of Obstetrics and Gynecology* **151**: 498–501.

Collings, CA, Curet, LB, Mullin JP (1983) Maternal and fetal responses to a maternal aerobic exercise program. *American Journal of Obstetrics and Gynecology* **145**: 702–7.

Condon JT (1987) Psychological and physical symptoms during pregnancy: a comparison of male and female expectant parents. *Journal of Reproductive and Infant Psychology* **5**: 207–13.

Cowlin A (1997) Women and exercise. In: Varney H, ed., *Varney's Midwifery*, 3rd edn. Boston, MA: Jones & Bartlett Publishers.

Cox JL, Holden JM, Sagovsky R (1987) Development of the 10- Item Edinburgh Postnatal Depression Scale. *British Journal of Psychiatry* **150**: 782–6.

Cox JL, Holden JM (1993) *The Prevention of Postnatal Depression Use and Misuse of the Edinburgh Postnatal Depression Scale. British Journal of Psychiatry Monographs.* Royal College of Psychiatrists: Gaskell Publications.

Crammer SR, Nieman DC, Lee JW (1991) The effects of moderate training on psychological well-being and mood state in women. *Journal of Psychosomatic Research* **35**: 437–49.

Crews DJ, Landers DM (1987) A meta-analytic review of aerobic fitness and reactivity to psychosocial stressors. *Medicine and Science in Sports and Exercise* **19**: 114–20.

Dale E, Mullinax KM, Bryan DH (1982) Exercise during pregnancy: Effects on the fetus. *Canadian Journal of Applied Sports Science* **7**: 98–103.

Department of Health (1994) *Guidance for NHS Health Records: A consultation paper.* London: HMSO.

Department of Health (1998) *Data Protection Act.* London: HMSO.

de Swiet M (1991a) The cardiovascular system. In: Hytten F, Chamberlain G, (Eds), *Clinical Physiology in Obstetrics.* Oxford: Blackwell Scientific Publications, pp. 3–38.

de Swiet M (1991b) The respiratory system. In: Hytten F, Chamberlain G, (Eds), *Clinical Physiology in Obstetric.* Oxford: Blackwell Scientific Publications, pp. 83–100.

Deutsch H (1947) *The Psychology of Women.* New York: Grune & Stratton.

Dick-Read G (1933) *Childbirth without Fear.* New York: Dell.

Dickinson RL (1895) Bicycling for women from the standpoint of the gynecologist. *American Journal of Obstetrics* **1**: 25.

Donnelly M (1988) *The American Victorian Woman: The myth and reality*. Westport, CT: Greenwood Press.

Douglas PS (1994) Cardiovascular disorders in women. In: Agostini R, ed., *Medical and Orthopedic Issues of Active and Athletic Women*. Philadelphia, PA: Hanley & Belfus.

Dressendorfer RH, Goodlin RC (1980) Fetal heart rate response to maternal exercise testing. *Physician and Sports Medicine* 8: 91–94.

Dunbar CC (1991) Practical use of ratings of perceived exertion in a clinical setting. *Sports Medicine* 16: 221–4.

Dumas GA, Reid JG (1997) Laxity of knee cruciate ligaments during pregnancy. *Journal of Orthopaedic, Sports Physical Therapy* 26: 2–6.

Durnin JVGA (1992) Physical activity levels: past and present. In: Norgan NG, (Ed) *Physical Activity and Health*. Cambridge: Cambridge University Press.

Duvekot JJ, Cheriex EC, Pieters FAA et al. (1993) Early pregnancy changes in hemodynamics and volume homeostasis are consecutive adjustments triggered by a primary fall in systemic vascular tone. *American Journal of Obstetrics and Gynecology* 169: 1382–92.

Duvekot JJ, Cheriex EC, Pieters FAA et al. (1995) Maternal volume homeostasis in early pregnancy in relation to fetal growth restriction. *Obstetrics and Gynecology* 85: 361–8.

Eccles A (1982) *Obstetrics and Gynaecology in Tudor and Stuart England*. London: Croom Helm Ltd.

Elliot SA, Rugg AJ, Watson JP, Brough DI (1983) Mood changes during pregnancy and after the birth of a child. *British Journal of Clinical Psychology* 22: 295–308.

Erikson M (1965) Relationships between psychological attitudes during pregnancy and complications of pregnancy, labour and delivery. In: *Proceedings of the Seventy-Third Annual Convention of the American Psychological Association*, Chicago, IL, pp. 213–15.

Erikson MT (1976) The relationship between psychological variables and specific complications of pregnancy, labour and delivery. *Journal of Psychosomatic Research* 20: 207–10.

Exodus I, Verse 19, *Old Testament, The Holy Bible*. Edinburgh: Collins Clear Type Press.

Fahlberg LL, Fahlberg LA (1996) Exercise programmes and the promotion of health In: Kerr J, Griffiths A, Cox T, eds, *Workplace Health: Employee fitness and exercise*. London: Taylor & Francis.

Fairbairn JS (1926) *Obstetrics*. London: Oxford Medical Publications.

Fiatarone M, O'Neill E, Ryan N et al. (1994) Exercise training and nutritional supplementation for physically frailty in very elderly people. *New England Journal of Medicine* 330: 1769–1775.

Fischman S, Rankin E, Soeken K, Lenz E (1986) Changes in sexual relationships in postpartum couples. *Journal of Obstetrics, Gynecology and Neonatal Nursing* Jan/Feb: 58–63.

Fox KR (1988) The self-esteem complex and youth fitness. *Quest* 40: 230–46.

Fox KR, Corbin CB (1989) The physical self perception profile: development and preliminary validation. *Journal of Sports Exercise Psychology* 11: 408–30.

Friederich M (1977) Psychological changes during pregnancy. *Contemporary Obstetrics and Gynecology* 9: 27–32.

Frisch RE, Wyashad G, Albright NL et al. (1987) Lower lifetime occurrence of breast cancer and cancers of the reproductive system among former college athletes. *International Journal of Fertility and Menopausal Studies* **32**(3) 217–25.

Galabin AL (1900) *A Manual of Midwifery*. London: Churchill.

Gannon L (1988) The potential role of exercise in the alleviation of menstrual disorders and menopausal symptoms: A theoretical synthesis of recent research. *Women and Health* **14**: 105–27.

Gaskill J (1992) *The Y-Plan Before and After Pregnancy: The complete pre- and postnatal fitness plan (video tape)*. London Central YMCA.

Gaskill J (1993) Exercise in pregnancy. *Journal of Association of Chartered Physiotherapists in Obstetrics and Gynaecology* **73**: 5–7.

Gaskill J (1994) No pause for pregnancy. *Practice Nurse* **1**: 207–15.

Gauthier MM (1986) Guidelines for exercise during pregnancy: Too little or too much? *The Physician and Sports Medicine* **14**: 162–9.

Gelis J (1991) *History of Childbirth*. Cambridge: Polity Press.

Gibbons LW, Blair SN, Cooper KH et al. (1983) Association between coronary heart disease risk factors and physical fitness in healthy adult women. *Circulation* **67**: 977–1002.

Glass SC, Knowlton RO, Becque MD (1992) Accuracy of RPE from graded exercise to establish exercise training intensity. *Medicine and Science in Sports and Exercise* **24**: 1303–7.

Glazer G (1980) Anxiety levels and concerns amongst pregnant women. *Research in Nursing and Health* **3**: 107–13.

Gordon H, Logue M (1985) Perineal muscle function after childbirth. *Lancet* **ii**: 123–125.

Gorski J (1985) Exercise during pregnancy: maternal and fetal response: A brief review. *Medicine and Science in Sports Exercise* **17**: 407–16.

Green CM (1892) Care of women in pregnancy. *Boston Medical and Surgical Journal* **CXXVI, 8**: 188.

Green JM (1990a) 'Who is unhappy after childbirth?' Antenatal and intrapartum correlates from a prospective study. *Journal of Reproductive and Infant Psychology* **8**: 175–83.

Green JM (1990b) Is the baby alright and other worries. *Journal of Reproductive and Infant Psychology* **8**: 225–6.

Green JM, Coupland VA, Kitzinger JV (1990) Expectations, experiences and psychological outcomes of childbirth: a prospective study of 825 women. *Birth* **17**: 15–24.

Griffiths A (1996) Employee exercise programmes: organisational and individual perspective. In: Kerr J, Griffiths A, Cox T, eds, *Workplace Health: Employee fitness and exercise*. London: Taylor & Francis, Chapter 1.

Grisso JA, Main DM, Chiu G, Synder ES, Holmes JM (1992 ) Effects of physical activity and lifestyle factors on uterine contraction frequency. *American Journal of Perinatology* **9**: 489–92.

Grossman FK, Eitchler LS, Winickoff SA (1980) *Pregnancy, Birth and Parenthood: Adaptation of mothers, fathers and infants*. San Francisco, CA: Jossey-Bass.

Guzman CA, Caplan R (1970) Cardiorespiratory responses to exercise during pregnancy. *American Journal of Obstetrics and Gynecology* **108**: 600–5.

Hale RW, Artal Mittlemark R (1991) Pregnancy in the elite athlete and professional athlete: A stepwise clinical approach. In: Artal Mittlemark R, Wiswell RA,

Drinkwater BL, (Eds), *Exercise in Pregnancy*, 2nd edn. Baltimore, MD: Williams & Wilkins, Chapter 20.

Halksworth G (1993) Exercise and pregnancy. In: Alexander J, Levy V, Roch S (Eds), *Midwifery Practice A research based approach*. Oxford: The Macmillan Press, Chapter 3.

Hall DC, Kaufmann DA (1987) Effects of aerobic and strength conditioning on pregnancy outcomes. *American Journal of Obstetrics and Gynecology* **157**: 1199–1203.

Hannah P, Adams D, Lee A, Glover V, Sandler M (1990) Early use of the Edinburgh Postnatal Depression Scale in the prediction of postnatal depression. Paper presented at the fifth International Conference of the Marce Society: Child Bearing and Mental Health, University of York.

Harris MB (1981) Women runners' views of running. *Perceptual Motor Skills* **53**: 295–402.

Harris B, Huckle P, Thomas R, Johns S, Fung H (1989) The use of self-rating scales to identify postnatal depression. *British Journal of Psychiatry* **154**: 813–17.

Harvey G (1950) *Eternal Eve*. Oxford: William Heinemann, Medical Books Ltd.

Hatch MC, Shu XO, Mclean DE et al. (1993) Maternal exercise during pregnancy, physical fitness and fetal growth. *American Journal of Epidemiology* **137**: 1105–14.

Haultain WFT, Fahmy ECF (1929) *Antenatal Care*. Edinburgh: Livingstone, Chapter 13.

Hauth JC, Gilstrap LC, Widmer K (1982) Fetal heart rate reactivity before and after maternal jogging during the third trimester. *American Journal of Obstetrics and Gynecology* **142**: 545–7.

Heardman H (1951) *Physiotherapy in Obstetrics and Gynaecology*. Edinburgh: Livingstone.

Heardman H (1959) *Relaxation and Exercise for Natural Childbirth*, 2nd edn. Edinburgh: E & S Livingstone.

Hedegaard M, Secher NJ, Wilcox AJ (1995) Standing at work and preterm delivery. *British Journal of Obstetrics and Gynecology* **102**: 198–206.

Heffernan AE (2000) Exercise and pregnancy in health care. *Nurse Practitioner* **25**(3): 42, 49, 53–6.

Henderson JS (1983) Effects of prenatal teaching program regeneration of the pubococcygeal muscle. *Journal of Obstetrics, Gynecology and Neonatal Nursing* **12**: 403–8.

Hirst J, Hewison J, Dowswell T, Baslington H, Warrilow J (1998) Antenatal care: What do women want? In: Clement S, ed., *Psychological Perspectives on Pregnancy and Childbirth*. Edinburgh: Churchill Livingstone, pp. 27–44.

Holbrook ML (1875) *Parturition Without Pain: A code of directions for escaping from the primal curse*. New York: Wood & Holbrook.

Homer CJ, Beresford SAA, James SA, Siegal E, Wilcox S (1990) Work related physical exertion and risk of preterm low birthweight delivery. *Paediatrics and Perinatology Epidemiology* **4**: 161.

Hon EH, Wohlgemuth R (1961) The electronic evaluation of fetal heart rate. The effect of maternal exercise. *American Journal of Obstetrics and Gynecology* **81**: 361–71.

Horns PN, Ratcliff LP, Leggett JC, Swanson MS (1996) Pregnancy outcomes among active and sedentary women. *Journal of Obstetric, Gynecologic, and Neonatal Nursing* **25**: 49–54.

Huch R, Erkkola R (1990) Pregnancy and exercise: exercise and pregnancy. A short review. *British Journal of Obstetrics and Gynaecology* **97**: 208–14.

Hughes JL (1984) Psychological effects of habitual aerobic exercise: A critical review. *Preventative Medicine* **13**: 66–78.

Hytten F, Chamberlain G, eds (1991) *Clinical Physiology in Obstetrics.* Oxford: Blackwell Scientific Publications.

Jackson MR, Gott P, Lye S et al. (1995) The effect of maternal aerobic exercise on human placental development: Placental volumetric composition and surface areas. *Placenta* **16**: 179–91.

Jamieson JL, Flood KR (1993) Experimental versus observational research methodologies In: Seraganian P, ed., *Exercise Psychology: The influence of exercise on psychological processes.* New York: John Wiley & Sons.

Jarrett JC, Spellacy WN (1983) Jogging during pregnancy: an improved outcome? *Obstetrics and Gynecology* **61**: 705–9.

Jovanovic L, Kessler A, Peterson CM (1988) Human maternal and fetal response to graded exercise. *Journal of Applied Physiology* **58**: 1719–22.

Kardel KR, Kase T (1998) Training in pregnant women: effects on fetal development and birth. *American Journal of Obstetrics and Gynecology* **178**: 280–6.

King JC, Butte NF, Bronstein MN et al. (1994) Energy metabolism during pregnancy: influence of maternal energy status. *American Journal of Clinical Nutrition* 59 (2): 439–45.

Klebanoff MA, Shiono PH, Carey CJ (1990) The effect of physical activity during pregnancy on preterm delivery, birth weight. *American Journal of Obstetrics and Gynecology* **163**: 1450–6.

Knuttgen HG, Emerson KJR (1974) Physiological response to pregnancy at rest and during exercise. *Journal of Applied Physiology* **36**: 549–53.

Koltyn KF, Schultes SS (1997) Psychological effects of an aerobic exercise session and a rest session following pregnancy. *Journal of Sports Medicine, Physical Fitness* **37**: 287–91.

Koniak-Griffin D (1994) Aerobic exercise, psychological well-being and physical discomforts during adolescent pregnancy. *Research in Nursing Health* **17**: 253–63.

Kramer MS (2000) Regular aerobic exercise during pregnancy. In: *The Cochrane Database of Systematic Reviews*, The Cochrane Library, Computer File (2): CD000189, Issue 4, Oxford: Update Software.

Kupla PJ, White BM, Visscher R (1987) Aerobic exercise in pregnancy. *American Journal of Obstetrics and Gynecology* **156**: 1395–1403.

Kumar R (1982) Neurotic disorders in childbearing women. In: Brockington IF, Kumar R, eds, *Motherhood and Mental Health.* London: Academic Press, pp. 71–118.

Kumar R, Brockington F (1988) *Motherhood and Mental Illness*, 2nd edn. London: Wright.

Kumar R, Robson K (1984) A prospective study of emotional disorders in childbearing women. *British Journal of Psychiatry* **144**: 35–47.

Kumar R, Robson KM, Smith AMR (1984) Development of self-administered questionnaire to measure maternal adjustment and maternal attitudes during pregnancy and after delivery. *Journal of Psychosomatic Research* **28**: 43–51.

La Forge R (1995) Exercise-associated mood alterations: A review of interactive neuro-biologic mechanisms. *Medicine, Exercise, Nutrition and Health* **4**: 17–32.

Lamaze F (1958) *Painless Childbirth*. London: Burke.

Lamb DR (1984) *Physiology of Exercise, Responses and Adaptations*, 2nd edn. New York: Macmillan.

Lamb KL, Brodie DA (1991) Leisure time physical activity as an estimate of physical fitness - a validity study. *Journal of Clinical Epidemiology* **44**: 41–52.

LaPorte REM, Montoye HL, Caspersen CJ (1985) Assessment of physical activity in epidemiological research: problems and prospects. *Public Health Reports* **100**: 131–46.

Lebrun CM (1994) Effects of the menstrual cycle and birth control pill on athletic performance. In: Agostini R, ed., *Medical and Orthopaedic Issues of Active and Athletic Women*. Philadelphia, Pa: Hanley, Belfus, pp. 78–91.

Lee G (1996) Exercise in pregnancy. *Modern Midwife* **6**(8): 28–33.

Leuzzi RA, Scoles KS (1996) Preconceptions counselling for the primary care physician. *Medical Clinicians North America* **80**: 337–374.

Lokey EA, Tran ZV, Wells CL, Myers BC, Tran AC (1991) Effects of physical exercise on pregnancy outcomes: a meta analytic review. *Medicine and Science in Sports and Exercise* **23**: 1234–9.

Lotgering FK, Gilbert RD, Longo LD (1983) Exercise response in pregnant sheep: consumption, uterine blood flow and blood volume. *Journal of Applied Physiology* **55**: 834–41.

Lotgering FK, Gilbert RD, Longo LD (1984) The interactions of exercise and pregnancy: A review. *American Journal of Obstetrics and Gynecology* **149**: 560–8.

Lotgering FK, Gilbert RD, Longo LD (1985) Maternal and fetal responses to exercise during pregnancy *Physiology Reviews* **65**: 1–36.

Loughlan CW (1995) Increasing health related physical activity in previously sedentary adults: a comparison of fitness testing and exercise consultation. PhD Thesis, University of Glasgow.

Lutter JM (1994) History of women in sports: societal issues. *Clinics in Sports Medicine* **13**: 263–7.

McCann L, Holmes DS (1984) Influence of aerobic exercise on depression. *Journal of Personality and Social Psychology* **46**: 1142–7.

Machin D, Campbell MJ (1991) *Statistical Tables for the Design of Clinical Trials*. Oxford: Blackwell.

McCrone KE (1988) *Sport and Physical Emancipation of English Women 1870–1914*. London: Routledge.

McGoldrick M, Carter E (1982) The family lifecycle. In: Walsh F, ed., *Normal Family Processes*. New York: Guilford Press.

McNair DM, Lorr N, Droppleman LF (1981) *Manual for the Profile of Mood States*. San Diego, CA: Education, Industrial Testing Service.

McNitt-Gray JL (1991) Biomechanics related to exercise in pregnancy. In: Artal Mittlemark R, Wiswell RA, Drinkwater BL (Eds) *Exercise in Pregnancy*, 2nd edn. Baltimore, MD: Williams & Wilkins, pp. 133–40.

Manders MA, Sonder GJ, Mulder EJ, Visser GH (1997) The effects of maternal exercise on fetal heart rate and movement patterns. *Early Human Development* **48**: 237–47.

Magness RR, Rosenfeld CR (1989) Local and systemic estradiol-17β: Effects on uterine and systemic vasodilation. *American Journal of Physiology* **256**: E536–E542.

Marcus, R, Drinkwater B, Dalsky G et al. (1992) Osteoporosis and exercise in women. *Medical Science and Sports Exercise* **24**(suppl): S301–S307.

Mayberry LJ, Smith M, Gill P (1992) Effect of exercise on uterine activity in the patient in preterm labour. *Journal of Perinatology* **12**: 354–8.

Misra DP, Stobino DM, Stashinko EE, Nagey DA, Nanda J (1998) Effects of physical activity on preterm labour. *American Journal of Epidemiology* **147**: 628–35.

Montgomery E (1969) *At Your Best for Birth and Later*, 3rd edn. Bristol: John Wright & Sons.

Morgan WP (1979) Anxiety reduction following acute physical activity. *Psychology Annals* **9**(3): 36–45.

Morgan WP (1985) Affective beneficence of vigorous physical activity. *Medicine and Science in Sports and Exercise* **17**: 94–100.

Morkvid S, Bo K (1996) The effect of postnatal exercises to strengthen the pelvic floor muscles. *Acta Obstetrica et Gynecologica Scandinavica* **75**: 382–5.

Morris JL, Pollard R, Everitt MG et al. (1980) Vigorous exercise in leisure time: a protection against coronary heart disease. *Lancet* ii: 1207–10.

Morris JN (1995) Exercise in the prevention of coronary heart disease: today's best buy in Public Health. *Medicine and Science in Sports and Exercise* **26**: 807–14.

Morris M (1936) *Maternity and Post-Operative Exercises*. London: Heinemann.

Moses J, Steptoe A, Mathews A, Edwards S (1989) The effects of exercise training on mental well being in the normal population: A controlled trial. *Journal of Psychosomatic Research* **33**: 47–61.

Mottola FM (1996) The use of animal models in exercise and pregnancy research. *Seminars in Perinatology* **20**: 222–31.

Mottola FM, Wolfe LA (1994) Active living and pregnancy. In: Quinney AH, Gauvin L, Wall TAE (Eds) cited in the *International Conference on Physical Activity, Fitness, Health*, pp. 311–338.

Munro Kerr MJ, Johnstone RW, Phillips MH (1954) *Historical Review of British Obstetrics and Gynaecology 1800–1950*. Edinburgh: E & S Livingstone Ltd.

Murray L, Carothers AD (1990) The validation of the Edinburgh Postnatal Depression Scale on a community sample. *British Journal of Psychiatry* **157**: 288–290.

Murray L, Cox JL (1990) Screening for depression during pregnancy with the Edinburgh Postnatal Depression Scale (EPDS). *Journal of Reproductive and Infant Psychology* **8**: 99–107.

Niven K (1992) *Psychological Care for Families Before, During, After Birth*. Oxford: Butterworth–Heinemann.

North TC, McCullagh P, Tran ZV (1990) Effect of exercise on depression. *Exercise and Sports Science Review* **18**: 379–415.

Oakley A (1992) *Social Support and Motherhood: A natural history of a research project*. Oxford: Blackwell.

Omar HA, Ramirez R, Gibson M (1995) Properties of a progesterone-induced relaxation in human placental arteries and veins. *Journal of Clinical Endocrinology and Metabolism* **80**: 307–73.

O'Neill ME, Cooper KA, Mills CM, Boyce ES, Hunyor SN (1992) Accuracy of Borg's ratings of perceived exertion in the prediction of heart rates during pregnancy. *British Journal of Sports Medicine* **26**: 121–4.

Osofsky JD, Osofsky HJ (1984) Psychological and developmental perspectives on expectant and new parenthood. In: Parke RD, Emde RN, McAdoo HP, Sackett GP, eds, *Review of Child Development Research*. Chicago: University of Chicago Press, pp. ??.

Parsons C (1994) Back care in pregnancy. *Modern Midwife* **4**(10): 16–19.

Pate R, Pratt M, Blair SN et al. (1995) Physical activity and public health. *Journal of the American Medical Association* **273**: 402–7.

Patrick K, Sallis JF, Long B et al. (1994) A new tool for encouraging activity: Project PACE. *Physician Sports Medicine* **22**: 45–52.

Pendergast JF (1896) The bicycle for women. *American Journal of Obstetrics* **34**: 245–53.

Pernoll ML, Metcalfe J, Schlenker TL, Welch JE, Matsumoto JA (1975) Oxygen consumption at rest and during exercise in pregnancy. *Respiratory Physiology* **25**: 285–93.

Pitt B (1977) Psychological aspects of pregnancy. *Midwife Health Visitor and Community Nurse* **13**: 137–9.

Pivarnik JM (1998) Potential effects of maternal physical activity on birthweight: brief review. *Medicine and Science in Sports and Exercise* **30**: 400–6.

Pivarnik JM, Lee W, Miller JF (1991) Physiological and perceptual responses to cycle and treadmill exercise during pregnancy. *Medicine and Science in Sports and Exercise* **23**: 470–5.

Pivarnik JM, Mauer MB, Ayres NA, Kirshon B, Dildy GA, Cotton DB (1994) Effects of chronic exercise on blood volume expansion and haemolytic indices during pregnancy. *Obstetrics and Gynecology* **83**: 265–9.

Plummer OK, Koh YO (1987) Effect of 'aerobics' on self concepts of college women. *Perceptual and Motor Skills* **65**: 271–5.

Pomerance JJ, Gluck L, Lynch VA (1974) Physical fitness in pregnancy: Its effect on pregnancy outcome. *American Journal of Obstetrics and Gynecology* **119**: 867–76.

Posner J, McCully K, Landsberg L et al. (1995) Physical determinants of independence in mature women. *Archives Physical Medical Rehabilitation* **76**: 373–80.

Price A (1993a) Altered body image in pregnancy and beyond. *British Journal of Midwifery* **1**: 142–6.

Price B (1993b) Women in labour: Body image, loss of control and coping behaviour. *Professional Care of Mother and Child* Nov/Dec: 280–2.

Price B (1996) Changing body image. *Modern Midwife* April: 12–15.

Quinton D, Rutter M, Rowland O (1976) An evaluation of an interview assessment of marriage. *Psychology and Medicine* **6**: 577–86.

Raglin JS (1990) Exercise and mental health: Beneficial and detrimental effects. *Sports Medicine* **9**: 323–9.

Raisanen I, Paatern H, Salminen KT et al. (1984) Pain and plasma beta endorphin level in labour. *Obstetrics and Gynecology* **64**: 783–6.

Randall M (1939) *Training for Childbirth*, 2nd edn. London: Churchill.

Raphael-Leff J (1991) *Psychological Processes of Childbearing*. London: Chapman & Hall.

Rauramo I, Andersson B, Laatikainen T (1982) Stress hormones and placental steroids in physical exercise during pregnancy. *British Journal of Obstetrics and Gynecology* **89**: 921–5.

Rees C (1997) *An Introduction to Research for Midwives.* Cheshire: Books for Midwives Press.

Riemann MK, Kanstrup Hansen I-L (2000) Effects on the foetus of exercise in pregnancy. *Scandinavian Journal of Medicine, Science in Sports* **10**: 12–19.

Robertson NRC (1993) *A Manual of Neonatal Intensive Care*, 3rd edn. London: Edward Arnold.

Rockhill B, Willett WC, Hunter DJ et al. (1998) Physical activity and breast cancer risk in a cohort of young women. *Journal of the National Cancer Institution* **90**: 1155–60.

Romen Y, Masaki DI, Mittlemark RA (1991) Physiological and endocrine adjustments to pregnancy. In: Mittlemark RA, Wiswell RA (Eds) *Exercise in Pregnancy*, 2nd edn. Baltimore, MD: Williams & Wilkins, pp. 9–29.

Rose NC, Haddow JE, Palomaki GE, Knight GJ (1991) Self-rated physical activity level during the second trimester and pregnancy outcome. *Obstetrics and Gynecology* **78**: 1078–80.

Roth DL, Holmes DS (1987) Influence of aerobic exercise training and relaxation training on physical and psychologic health following stressful life events. *Psychosomatic Medicine* **49**: 355–65.

Royal College of Physicians (1993) *Promoting Physical Activity: Partnerships for Action.* Faculty of Public Health Medicine Bulletin Number 32.

Schrier RW, Briner VA (1991) Peripheral arterial vasodilation hypothesis of sodium and water retention in pregnancy: implications for pathogenesis of pre-eclampsia. *Obstetrics and Gynecology* **77**: 632–9.

Scott-Heyes G (1984) Marital adaptation during pregnancy and after childbirth. *Reproductive and Infant Psychology* **1**: 18–29.

Scottish Office Home and Health Department (1992) *Scotland's Health: A challenge to us all.* Edinburgh: HMSO.

Sharp DJ (1989) Emotional disorders during pregnancy and the puerperium: longitudinal prospective study in primary care. *Marce Soc Bulletin* Spring.

Sharp C (1993) Physiological aspects of pregnancy and exercise. *Journal of the Association of Chartered Physiotherapy in Obstetrics and Gynaecology* **73**: 8–13.

Shephard AM (1983) Management of urinary incontinence - prevention or cure? *Physiotherapy* **69**: 109 - 110.

Sibley L, Ruhling RO, Cameron-Foster J, Christensen C, Bolen T (1981) Swimming and physical fitness during pregnancy. *Journal of Nurse-Midwifery* **26**: 3–12.

Sieber JE (1992) *Planning Ethically Responsible Research.* London: Sage.

Simkin AJ, Ayalon J, Leichter J (1987) Increased tabular bone density on to bone loading exercise on post menopausal osteoporotic women. *Calcified Tissue International* **40**: 59–63.

Slavin JL, Lutter JM, Cushman S, Lee V (1988) Pregnancy and exercise. In: Puhl J, Brown CH, Voy RO (Eds) *Sport Science Perspectives for Women.* Champaign, IL: Human Kinetics, pp. 151–60.

Sleep J, Grant A (1987) Pelvic floor exercises in postnatal care. *Midwifery* **3**: 158–64.

Smith E, Smith KA, Gilligan C (1990) Exercise, fitness and osteoporosis. In: Bouchard C, Shephard RJ, Stephens T (Eds) *Physical Activity, Fitness and Health*. Champaign, IL: Human Kinetics Publishers.

Smith SB (1979) *The People's Health 1830–1910*. London: Croom Helm, pp. 26–7.

Snaith RP, Constantapoulas AA, Jardine MU, McGuffin P (1978) A clinical scale for the self assessment of irritability. *British Journal of Psychiatry* 132: 164–71.

Snooks SJ, Setchell M, Swash M, Henry MM (1984) Injury to innervation of pelvic floor sphincter musculature in childbirth. *Lancet* ii: 546–50.

South-Paul JE, Rajagopal KR, Tenholder MF (1988) The effect of participation in a regular exercise program upon aerobic capacity during pregnancy. *Obstetrics and Gynecology* 71: 175–9.

Stephens T (1988) Physical activity and mental health in the United States and Canada: Evidence from four populations studies. *Preventative Medicine* 17: 35–47.

Steptoe A (1992) Physical Activity and psychological well-being. In: Norgan NG (Ed) *Physical Activity and Health*. London: Cambridge University Press, Chapter 15.

Steptoe A, Edwards S, Moses J, Mathews A (1989) The effects of exercise training on mood and perceived coping ability in anxious adults from the general population. *Psychosomatic Research* 33: 537–47.

Stern DM, Burnett CWF (1958) *A Modern Practice of Obstetrics*, 2nd edn. London: Ballière Tindall & Cox.

Sternfield B (1997) Physical activity and pregnancy outcomes. Review and recommendations. *Sports Medicine* 23: 22–47.

Sternfield B, Quesenberry CB, Eskenazi B et al. (1995) Exercise during pregnancy and pregnancy outcome. *Medicine and Science and Sports and Exercise* 27: 634–40.

Strang VR, Sullivan PL (1985) Body image, attitude during pregnancy and postpartum period. *Journal of Obstetrics, Gynecology and Neonatal Nursing* July/Aug: 332–6.

Sweet B, Tiran D (Eds) (1997) *Mayes Midwifery A Textbook for Midwives*. London: Ballière Tindall.

Tanji JL (2000) The benefits of exercise for women. *Clinics in Sports Medicine* 19: 175–83.

Thirlaway K, Benton D (1996) Exercise and mental health: the role of activity and fitness. In: Kerr, J, Griffiths A, Cox T (1996) *Workplace Health: Employee fitness and exercise*. London: Taylor & Francis, Chapter 4.

Thomas JR, Nelson JK (1990) *Research Methods in Physical Activity*, 2nd edn. Champaign, IL: Human Kinetics Publications.

Thune I, Brenn T, Lund E et al. (1997) Physical activity and risk of breast cancer. *New England Journal of Medicine* 36: 1269–75.

Tobin SM (1967) Carpal tunnel syndrome in pregnancy. *American Journal of Obstetrics and Gynecology* 23: 493.

Ueland K, Novy MJ, Peterson EN, Metcalfe J (1969) Maternal cardiovascular dynamics IV: The influence of gestational age on the maternal cardiovascular response to posture and exercise. *American Journal of Obstetrics and Gynecology* 104: 856–64.

United Kingdom Central Council for Nursing, Midwifery, Health Visiting (1996) *Guidelines for Professional Practice*. London: UKCC.

Ussher J (1993) *The Psychology of the Female Body*. London: Routledge.

Valancogne G, Galaup JP (1993) Rehabilitation during pregnancy and in the post-partum period (Review). *French Gynecology and Obstetrics* **88**: 498–508.

Varrassi G, Bazzano C, Edwards TW (1989) Effects of physical activity on maternal plasma beta endorphin levels and pain perception of labour pain. *American Journal of Obstetrics and Gynecology* **160**: 707–12.

Vaughan K (1942) The expanding pelvis. *British Medical Journal* i: 786.

Vaughan K (1951) *Exercise before Childbirth*. London: Faber & Faber Ltd, pp. 12–30.

Veille JC, Hohimer AR, Burry K, Speroff L (1985) The effects of uterine activity on the last eight weeks of pregnancy. *American Journal of Obstetrics and Gynecology* **151**: 727–30.

Vertinsky P (1990) *The Eternally Wounded Woman. International Studies in the History of Sport*. Manchester: Manchester University Press.

Wallace AM, Boyer DB, Dan A, Holm K (1986) Aerobic exercise, maternal self-esteem, and physical discomforts during pregnancy. *Journal of Nurse Midwife* **31**: 255–62.

Wang TW, Apgar BS (1998) Exercise during pregnancy. *American Family Physician* **57**: 1846–57.

Ward A, Morgan WP (1984) Adherence patterns of healthy men and women enrolled in an adult exercise program. *Journal of Cardiac Rehabilitation* **4**: 143–52.

Watson JP, Elliot SA, Rugg AH, Brough DI (1984) Psychiatric disorder in pregnancy and in the first postnatal year. *British Journal of Psychiatry* **144**: 453–62.

Watson WJ, Katz VL, Hackney AC, Gall MM, McMurray RG (1991) Fetal responses to maximal swimming and cycling exercise during pregnancy. *Obstetrics and Gynecology* **77**: 382–6.

Webb KA, Wolfe LA, McGrath MJ (1994) Effects of acute and chronic maternal exercise on fetal heart rate. *Journal of Applied Physiology* **77**: 2207–10.

Wells CL (1991) *Women, Sport and Performance: A physiological perspective*, 2nd edn. Champaign, IL: Human Kinetics.

Wenger NK (1998) Coronary heart disease in women. In: Wallis LA, ed., *Textbook of Women's Health*. Philadelphia, PA: Lippincott-Raven, pp. 329–340.

Wheatley S (1998) Psychological support in pregnancy. In: Clement S (Ed) *Psychological Perspectives on Pregnancy and Childbirth*. Edinburgh: Churchill Livingstone, pp. 45–60.

Wolfe LA, Ohtake PJ, Mottola MF, McGrath MJ (1989a) Physiological interaction between pregnancy and aerobic exercise. In: Pandorf KB (Ed) *Exercise and Sports Science Reviews*, volume 17. Baltimore, MD: Williams & Wilkins: pp. 295–351.

Wolfe LA, Hall P, Webb KA, Goodman L, Monga M, McGrath MJ (1989b) Prescription of aerobic exercise during pregnancy. *Sports Medicine* **8**: 273–301.

Wolkind S, Zajicek E (1981) *Pregnancy: A psychological and social study*. London: Academic Press.

Young J (1940) Relaxation of the pelvis joints in pregnancy, pelvic arthropathy of pregnancy. *Journal of Obstetrics and Gynaecology of the British Empire* **47**: 493–6.

Zaharieva E (1972) Olympic participation by women. Effects on pregnancy and childbirth. *Journal of the American Medical Association* **221**: 992–5.

Zajicek E (1981) The experience of being pregnant. In: Wolkind S, Zajicek E (Eds) *Pregnancy: A psychological and social study*. New York: Grune & Stratton, Academic Press.

Zeanah M, Schlosser SP (1993) Adherence to ACOG guidelines on exercise during pregnancy: effect on pregnancy outcome. *Journal of Obstetrics and Gynecology and Neonatal Nursing* **22**: 329–35.

Zuspan FP, Cibils LA, Pose IV (1962) Myometrial and cardiovascular responses to alterations in plasma epinephrine and norepinephrine. *American Journal of Obstetrics and Gynecology* **84**: 841–51.

# Index

Printed and bound by CPI Group (UK) Ltd, Croydon, CR0 4YY

09/06/2025

14685974-0001